Mastering Statistics

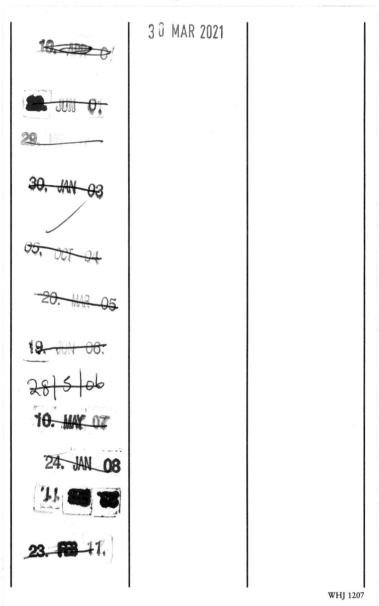

Mastering Statistics

A GUIDE FOR HEALTH SERVICE PROFESSIONALS AND RESEARCHERS

Kelvin Jordan*, Bie Nio Ong* & Peter Croft[†]

*Centre for Health Planning and Management,
Keele University
Staffordshire, UK

[†]Industrial and Community Health Research Centre,
Keele University
Staffordshire, UK

Stanley Thornes (Publishers) Ltd

First published in 1998 by
Stanley Thornes (Publishers) Ltd
Ellenborough House
Wellington Street
CHELTENHAM
GL50 1YW
United Kingdom

98 99 00 01 02 / 10 9 8 7 6 5 4 3 2 1

A catalogue record for this book is available from the British Library

ISBN 0–7487–3325–6

Typeset by Northern Phototypesetting Co. Ltd, Bolton, Lancs.
Printed and bound in Great Britain
by T.J. International Ltd, Padstow, Cornwall

In memory of Joseph

CONTENTS

ACKNOWLEDGEMENTS

We have many people to thank for their help in the production of this book. Firstly, to everyone who participated in the limiting long-term illness study and the hospital pre-assessment satisfaction study, we owe a great deal of thanks.

We also want to thank those who offered helpful comments and advice on the book; including Peter Jones who is Professor of Statistics at Keele University; Tony Wayte, List Development Manager in Health Sciences at Stanley Thornes, and the anonymous referee who provided a number of useful suggestions.

As well as this, we thank SPSS (UK) Ltd for allowing us to use SPSS for Windows as the main analysis tool in this text, and the Medical Outcomes Trust for allowing us to use the Short Form-36 in the limiting long-term illness study in this book. The contact details of the Medical Outcomes Trust are in Appendix C.

We are very grateful to Barbara Goodenough for her work in getting the book in a fit state to be sent to the publishers, and to Paul Trinder in helping out with some of the artwork.

Finally, we thank all those who have endured living, working and socialising with us during the writing of this book. They may now breathe a sigh of relief!

1 INTRODUCTION

1.1 WHY ANOTHER BOOK ON STATISTICS?

Health services research has risen to (renewed) prominence in many western countries over the last decade, and is increasingly seen as making an important contribution to understanding the provision and distribution of health services in relation to the needs of populations, and the way in which health care is organised and used. A large number of definitions have been provided as to what health services research actually is (Crombie and Davies, 1996) but in this book we use the definition from the Select Committee on Science and Technology (1988) which states that it is 'all strategic and applied research concerned with the health needs of the community as a whole, including the provision of services to meet those needs'. This definition is consistent with a broader definition of health as including not only physical, but also psychological, social and economic well-being which allows for a better understanding of the connection between health need and the use and effectiveness of specific interventions and services. The questions concerning targeting and priority setting, effectiveness and efficiency can be included within the HSR remit. Furthermore, the approach affords a contextual study of health need looking at the important areas such as inequalities in health and variations in the distribution and uptake of health services. This means that the territory of HSR is very wide, including the study of patterns of health and illness (e.g. Illsley and LeGrand, 1987; Benzeval et al., 1995), effectiveness of care (e.g. Jennett, 1988; Haines and Jones, 1994), diffusion of clinical innovation (e.g. Hoare, 1992; Banta and Vondeling, 1994); resource availability and priority setting (e.g. Allen, 1993; Malek, 1994).

With HSR ranging over such a wide territory it is no surprise that a broad methodological approach has to be adopted, including both qualitative and quantitative research. We will not repeat the by now well-known discussions surrounding the strengths and weaknesses of each (see e.g. Bryman, 1988; Brannen, 1992; Ong, 1993) and the appropriate application of the different theoretical and operational principles. While a multitude of methodologies may be adopted, many studies require a quantitative basis to the empirical data collection and analysis, and most researchers encounter the need to use statistical methods in their research design. It is at this point that the researcher turns to the statistical literature, and numerous books are available for both the novice and the experienced researcher. However, the majority of the books adopt a technical approach to statistics and often frighten the not statistically trained researcher. A small number of books address the design questions (e.g. Cartwright and Seale, 1990) or adopt a case study approach (Rees, 1994). They address some of the doubts of the researcher lacking statistical confidence but often do not offer graduated guidance linking realistic examples with specific statistical problems and possible solutions. It is precisely at this interface that we intend to address the reader: through a step-by-step journey through real-life research projects we present examples where statistical methods are required to address research questions. We will explain the reasons for selecting specific methods, their limitations and advantages, the technical execution of procedures and the interpretation of the results. By using actual research, most of which we have carried out ourselves, we can illustrate the beauty and the pitfalls of using statistics in a concrete manner. Theoretical and technical issues can be addressed through this pragmatic approach, rather than trying to fit the reality of messy research to ideal-typical statistics. We assume that readers will use computers, so statistical formulae will be kept to a minimum.

1.2 THE MAIN EXAMPLES

1.2.1 The limiting long-term illness study

The main study used in this book illustrating statistical issues is the research project that the three authors have undertaken examining limiting long-term illness in a general practice population in the West Midlands area of the UK. This study follows a tradition of research into patterns of health and illness, and in particular work pertaining to chronic illness. Heurtin-Roberts and Becker (1993, p. 281) define chronic illnesses as 'health conditions that can be managed but not cured, chronic illnesses have ongoing or periodic symptoms that interfere with daily life'. This definition is very close to the one used in the British Census, where limiting long-term illness (LLI) is defined as follows: 'a long-term illness, health problem or handicap which limits the daily activities or work that a person can do' (Dale and Marsh, 1993). In the national Census, this question is asked of all people in households and communal establishments and is not concerned with specific illnesses, health problems, handicaps or disabilities. Furthermore, it includes the added clause that problems due to old age should also be reported.

The information yielded by the health-related question in a census allows for national comparisons on LLI by age, economic position, ethnic group, household composition and housing characteristics. Thus, it provides an important basis for the establishment of indicators of need for health and social services for people with LLI. The national data offer the background for more local studies, such as the one we use in this book, and provide opportunities for tests of reliability and the setting of a broader context.

There has been a lot of discussion about the possible bias of the LLI question, such as, for example, the subjectivity of people's self-assessment. Charlton and colleagues (1994) argue that the response bias will not vary from one area of the country to another, implying that the prime objective of the LLI question is to allow comparisons between areas and localities. Further debate has surrounded the question as to whether the LLI question picks up more elderly people as a result of the specific addition of problems due to old age. Benzeval and Judge (1993) found that this was true for people in the age group 75 years and older, but that the rates fell for both sexes in the younger age groups. While these reservations should not be underestimated (see Jordan, 1996 for a fuller review) it is important to realise that the LLI question has produced better results than tested census questions on disability and ill-health, and has been consistent with the results obtained from other national surveys such as the General Household Survey. It clearly establishes the relationship between the presence of an LLI and the use of health services, and as such has value for health planners and policy-makers who require measures of health need of a population.

In the 1991 census 6.67 million people reported an LLI, representing 12% of the total resident population in the UK. The rate of LLI increased with rising age for both men and women, but there were great variations between different parts of the country. The local differences were very clear when looking at the West Midlands, and in particular the Stoke-on-Trent area. Forrest and Gordon (1995) have constructed a 'league table' of all districts in England, in which Stoke-on-Trent occupies the ninth place with 32.6% of households containing at least one person with an LLI. Standardized for age and sex (i.e. removing the effects of different age and sex structures of the districts) the ratio for Stoke-on-Trent is 136.4 compared to the national (mean) average of 100, while the neighbouring district of Newcastle-under-Lyme fares better with a ratio of 112.8 but is still well above the national (mean) average. The high local rates of ill-health prompted the local health authority and general practitioners to discuss with the three authors the possibility of a study to analyse this issue in more depth. The design for the study will be discussed in more detail in the second chapter.

In most western countries the population is ageing as a result of improvements in general living conditions. Advances in clinical medicine such as the treatment of secondary infections and the effectiveness of drugs and surgery, improving the management of many chronic illnesses, have increased the life expectancy of people suffering from diseases such as diabetes, myocardial infarction, epilepsy and multiple sclerosis (Gerhardt, 1990). The implications are that the increased longevity is not always accompanied by good health and chronic illnesses can become the main feature of life in later years. The World Health Organisation predicts that the incidence of cancers, circulatory diseases and diabetes will rise dramatically in the next two decades largely as a result of an ageing population combined with environmental and behavioural factors (WHO, 1997). Consequently, the importance of knowing the patterns and experiences of LLI is becoming more poignant, especially when predicting future care needs.

Bebbington (1988) carried out a study in England and Wales calculating the expectation for a life without disability. While his formula was not wholly perfect, his prediction was that around 80% of life could be lived without disability, but for people of 65 years and over this dropped to only half of their remaining life. He also hypothesized that people are experiencing longer periods of chronic disability. The expectation that the number of people suffering from an LLI will increase, and that their treatments will be maintained over longer periods of time and often also involve more complex regimes, sharpens the mind of health planners and policy-makers. The needs of these populations have to be well understood in order to devise interventions that improve their quality of life and are cost-effective. Health and social care providers focus both on the professional care aspects and on the experience of illness of the sufferers. Increasingly sophisticated measurements of disease are being developed and the clinical diagnosis and treatment are often being supplemented by assessments of effectiveness and quality of life. Standardized instruments can now be used alongside diagnostic criteria and either disease-specific instruments such as, for example, the Arthritis Impact Measurement Scale are used, or more general health profile measures such as the Short Form-36 (for a detailed discussion of instruments see Bowling, 1994, 1997). The administration of these formal instruments assists in understanding the impact of specific treatments on the quality of life, even though this can only be a 'snapshot' and is often limited to more functional aspects of the illness experience.

The perspective of the people suffering from LLI is a more complex area of research because it has to be seen within the social and cultural context within which sufferers live. Each society operates with its own set of values about normality, which includes normal physical functioning, cultural norms about membership of social groups, appearance and behaviour. Chronic illness threatens some of the ideas about normality and many individuals suffering with an LLI are excluded and marginalized from mainstream society because they cannot exercise their normal, daily activities and fulfil their expected social roles. This process of stigmatization (Goffman, 1963) affects both chronically ill people as a group and the individuals within them and profoundly colours the way they experience their ill-health. Understanding those experiences is important if we are to assess whether support from statutory health and social care agencies responds to those experiences and allows individuals to participate in society as 'normal' people.

In the research study used in this book all three aspects of LLI have been examined: the broader patterns of LLI at national and local level, using the census question on LLI and a standardized instrument, the Short Form-36 (SF-36); the clinical assessments and their (mis)match with people's self-assessed health status; and in-depth analysis of people's experiences of ill-health. These three perspectives inform each other and allow for a more complex understanding of LLI. In this book we will, however, only discuss the work carried out in the first two surveys using the census question on LLI and the SF-36 because they provide the laboratory for the statistical explanations (for information about the other two parts of the study see Jordan, 1996, Jordan et al., 1997 and Ong et al., forthcoming). The first survey involved sending the LLI census question to a sample of patients registered at one general practice; the second survey asked everyone who reported an LLI in the first survey to complete the SF-36, and a similar number of people who reported no LLI were selected to complete the SF-36 also as a comparison. The idea was that the two groups should have similar characteristics in terms of the breakdown of their age, sex and area of residence. More details of the study will be given as we progress through the life of the study.

1.2.2 The user feedback study

The increased emphasis on quality in health care has highlighted the need for providers to systematically assess this. One of the main mechanisms used in North America and western Europe is through user (patient) feedback. The development of surveys and questionnaires has been widespread, but the information gleaned from this sort of study has been extremely variable. Often the design has been flawed, questionnaires vague, samples unrepresentative and so on. Bruster and colleagues (1994) argued that many user surveys have been of little use to health care managers in helping them to locate or solve problems. Instead, they designed a detailed questionnaire asking people about their care and what actually happened during their hospital stay, covering issues such as communications, patient preferences, emotional support, physical comfort, pain management, education, family participation, discharge planning and financial information. Rather than focusing on the traditional satisfaction-type questions, this detailed approach allowed for a better understanding of the form and nature of specific problems, which can then be addressed by managers.

We adapted the approach by Bruster and colleagues to investigate the introduction of nurse-led preoperative assessment in a UK general hospital. Preoperative assessment was introduced as a response to a number of policy changes: first, the pressure to reduce hospital waiting lists. Better preoperative organization, targeted patient preparation and a reduction in ward administration were some of the benefits of the assessment clinic that were cited. Second, the reduction of junior doctors' hours and the shortening of specialist medical training led to experiments in nurse substitution (Dowling *et al.*, 1995). Third, patient pressure created the awareness of the importance of good information and communication and Ley (1988), for example, argued that this led to quicker and less stressful recovery. The time afforded in the preoperative assessment clinic contributed significantly to the quality of information received.

The purpose of our study was to assess the benefits (and problems) associated with the introduction of a nurse-led preoperative assessment clinic on a surgical ward. The questionnaire used by Bruster *et al.* (1994) was adapted for this specific purpose by focusing on the preoperative visit, including questions such as communication, the role of the nurse and the content and impact of the information given.

The nurse sees on average 11–14 patients per week in the

preoperative assessment clinic. A random sample was drawn from those attending over an 8-month period consisting of 25 men and 25 women. A total of 27 people were aged 55 years and over. The most common problems they had were cholecystectomy (9), hernia (9), bowel/colon (7) and breast operations (6).

Interviews were arranged directly between the hospital's Audit Department and the respondents. All interviews took place in the patients' homes at a mutually convenient time. The questionnaire schedules were filled in during the interview, augmented with any additional comments, given that the duration of the interviews was between 45 and 60 minutes. The precoded questions were analysed using the Microsoft Excel spreadsheet and SPSS for Windows, while the open-ended questions were grouped retrospectively according to themes.

1.2.3 The randomized controlled trial

We have chosen to include a discussion of the randomized controlled trial (RCT) because it is considered the backbone of clinical scientific studies and uses key statistical approaches in its data analysis. We will draw on a practical example, such as the treatment of asthma in a primary care setting, but the issues discussed pertain to RCTs in general. The key principles of the RCT design will be explained and the problems relating to bias will be discussed in considerable detail. This is important not only in order to avoid these difficulties but also because this will help you to see probability statistics in practice. Different models for RCTs are dealt with in this chapter, outlining their specific use. The null hypothesis will be revisited because it has a specific application in the RCT, as well as the concept of the odds ratio.

It is important to understand the limitations of the RCT when there are, for example, multiple goals or when the input cannot be controlled. Hunter (1993) points out that RCTs only work under specific circumstances, including unambiguous specification of the objective of interventions, foreseeable and measurable control over both the nature and the quality of the input, exclusion of external influences and uncontroversial measurement of success along a single dimension. Thus, like with other methodologies, the strengths and weaknesses of RCTs will be addressed as part of the overall discussion of the statistical issues relating to this approach.

1.3 THE LOGIC AND STRUCTURE OF THE BOOK

This book intends to take the reader through the most common issues when using statistical methods in health services research. The real-life examples of our own LLI study, epidemiological and nursing research should help in understanding the relevance and application of statistics in straightforward language. We really hope to demystify statistics and demonstrate their added value in the design, execution and analysis of empirical research studies.

The second chapter discusses the importance of good research design. This is often the invisible work that goes on before a research project starts, but is the crucial stage for ensuring that the planned research actually delivers what it intends to do. Thus, the discussion will cover some general design considerations before applying them to the specific example of survey research. The main phases of a survey are outlined, with the key design decisions that have to be made at each juncture.

The third and fourth chapters cover technical issues such as sampling and questionnaire design. While there are numerous texts covering these topics, we will provide a review of the main issues and the pitfalls and offer practical guidance for how to avoid them. Reference will be made to more in-depth literature, but with these two chapters you should be able to confidently make a start on your own project.

The following chapters focus on the question of what to do with the data collected. The design phase has clearly defined the purpose of the research and the statistical analysis has to be aligned to that purpose. First, Chapter 5 presents an overview of what is available in terms of computer packages and what their respective strengths and weaknesses are. Then, the mundane tasks of data entry, assessing the quality of the data and beginning to order the material are the next steps. Summarizing and ordering the data is covered in Chapter 6, discussing averages, measures of the spread (or variability) of the data and its distribution.

Basically, the first section of this book introduces you to the rules for collecting and summarizing data, while the second part of the book enters more complicated territory including the examination of the range of measures available to the analyst. Before you start on these chapters, we provide you with a short introduction in Chapter 7 which goes over what you have learned so far (and you can then check whether you have really grasped the main concepts) before outlining what lies ahead. You will not necessarily need everything in Chapters 8–10 because it depends very much on the scope and detail of the research you are, or want to be, involved in. Therefore, we have inserted a 'navigation map' which will help you to make choices, depending on the sorts of question you are asking or hypotheses you want to test, the type of data at your disposal or the analytical depth required. We promised to make statistics more transparent, which does not mean that we can always avoid the difficult bits, but we can help you decide the level of complication you want to get involved in. Thus, use Chapter 7 to work out your route through the remainder of the book.

Chapters 8–10 draw inferences from the data and begin to do the analytical work, relating your data to the wider population from which you extracted it. A range of tests and their associated conventions are explained, which are then pulled together in Chapter 10 with the discussion of the relationships between variables, leading to drawing conclusions on the basis of your statistical calculations.

Chapter 11 is devoted to the RCT, and we discuss the principles underlying the RCT and its central position within clinical research. The important question of bias in RCTs will be addressed as there are many sources of bias relating to the individuals involved, the context and the researchers themselves. It is vital that these sources of bias are understood at the outset so that the study design can be adjusted to counteract these. The main statistical applications in the RCT are outlined, including significance testing, confidence intervals, randomization strategies and so on. Within the scope of this book we can only deal with the broad principles and common pitfalls of the RCT and we refer to more detailed books on RCTs for those readers who want to actually design their own study.

Writing research reports is an essential part of the research endeavour because this ensures that your work can be disseminated. The readers of the report are often not statistically proficient and it helps if the report is written in a 'user-friendly' manner. In the final chapter we will offer suggestions as to the logic of how research findings can be presented making the most of the statistical evidence accumulated over the course of the project while not overburdening a report. Clarity and simplicity will help with the dissemination of findings, which, certainly in the field of HSR, is increasingly emphasized. There are a whole host of potential users, including planners, policy-makers, care-providers and users who would like to have access to scientifically solid but relevant material and we propose that sufficient attention needs to be paid to the production of such documents.

Each chapter provides guidance on further reading and a few helpful hints will be scattered throughout the text. Overall, we hope that by using this book you feel that statistics are useful rather than scary, and that they will find a place in your current or future research projects.

2 RESEARCH DESIGN AND SURVEYS

2.1 WHAT IS RESEARCH DESIGN?

Imagine that you are giving a dinner party. It is the first time that your boss or a colleague is coming to your house and you want to prepare something to impress him or her, tasteful but not ostentatious. You need also to have sufficient time to entertain your guest when s/he arrives and not be frazzled by complicated last-minute preparations. You think the best thing is to have a cold starter, which can be prepared ahead, a main meal that can all be set out and requires only heating up and a quick stir-fry, and a dessert ready to serve without any further work. The tastes have to be contrasting and interesting and the whole should leave the diners satisfied but not full up. Once you have set all these parameters to achieve your purpose, i.e. to impress but not overstate, you can consult your cookbooks for the technicalities of actual recipes that fit the bill.

In contrast, you could be planning a dinner party for a group of old friends who just want to have a good time together. You would be most likely to organize a type of meal where people have to pass round dishes and share with each other. The dessert has to be spectacular, as the crowning glory of the whole get-together. Thus, you want to have lots of strong-tasting food and plenty of drink to wash it down with, enhancing the high spirits. Your cookbooks will guide you in the direction of an Indonesian rice table or a Mexican tortilla feast.

Looking at these two examples you see that the hardest work lies in the thinking about what you want to achieve: creating or reinforcing a good impression with your boss or having a lovely party with your friends. Your design of a meal to fulfil the differing objectives requires careful planning of the various stages and how they fit together to make a coherent whole. Considerations of resources such as skills, time and money play an important role in settling for a final design. The consultation of the cookbooks is the easier bit as you can then assess recipes against the criteria you have set out in your design.

What are the parallels with research design? The design of a research project is like the design of a menu, somewhat of an artistic creation. The purpose of research is often set for the researcher by those who commission a piece of work, but they leave the interpretation of that purpose and the way in which it should be investigated to the researcher. This person is expected to provide ideas and coherent plans of how to tackle the research question, often refining or even changing the original question. Thus, design is not a purely technical exercise – even though technical knowledge forms an important part of the scientific basis – but a rather more creative exercise allowing the researcher to imprint his or her own 'style' (Hakim, 1987, p. 1). The thought processes associated with design are theoretically informed, but also have a strong pragmatic element and

Hakim's (1987) description of what design is reflects this: 'Design deals primarily with aims, uses, purposes, intentions and plans within the practical constraints of location, time, money and availability of staff' (p. 1).

Another important issue in research design is the need to make choices (Ong, 1993). There is no ideal multipurpose research method and consequently researchers must evaluate the strengths and weaknesses of different methods in relation to the purpose to be achieved. These choices can be informed by external forces, e.g. the specific demands of sponsors, or by internal considerations such as available skills and technical back-up, the logic of the whole research programme or the timing of the research. It is imperative that the choices made are explicitly stated in order to allow readers or users of the research to understand the considerations behind the design and why certain alternatives were excluded. To some extent it is also a sort of protection for the researcher because the transparency of the thinking process guards against charges of narrow-mindedness or bias. This is increasingly important in an era where researchers are more overtly held accountable for their research.

The clarity and appropriateness of the research design are key to convincing sponsors that the research has value to them. Furthermore, it helps to focus your own thinking on the presentation of results, their dissemination and implementation alongside other questions such as the cost-effectiveness and efficiency of your design. A good design will also involve setting timetables and project deadlines, and nowadays sponsors like to see a number of milestones flagged up within the design. This is where intermediate analyses at crucial points can be integrated within the overall design, and you need to select appropriate methods to deliver those midterm goals. While a beautifully designed research project is no guarantee that you will be able to deliver what you have set out to do – or have been asked to do – it provides a strong framework for a range of research decisions while keeping you focused on the end result.

2.2 WHAT IS A SURVEY?

The survey represents one of the prime study types used in the social sciences and there is an extensive literature on the subject. The classic by Moser and Kalton (1971) is one of the most often quoted and they include a wide range of studies within this type, such as poverty surveys, planning surveys, government social surveys, market research, population surveys and academic surveys. Baker (1991) argues that because of the wide range of studies classed under the heading of surveys it is better to provide a number of indicators of what surveys are concerned with:

- fact finding;
- by asking questions;
- of persons representative of the population of interest;

- to determine attitudes and opinions; and
- to help understand and predict behaviour (p. 85).

This definition fits within the more conceptual approach taken by Marsh (1982), who states that, within a survey:

- systematic measurements are made over a series of cases yielding a rectangle of data;
- the variables in the matrix are analysed to see if they show any patterns;
- the subject matter is social (p. 6).

Cartwright (1983) in her review of health surveys makes the explicit link with theory when she says that 'surveys are essentially a research tool by which facts can be ascertained, theories confirmed or refuted, ideas explored and values identified and illuminated. So the sorts of questions with which surveys are concerned relate to the distribution and association of facts and attitudes' (p. 1). The theoretical foundation is important because the survey should contribute to a better understanding of what people think and what they do, and sociological theories help in interpreting the facts ascertained through the survey approach.

Fink (1995), in her introduction to the *Survey Kit*, provides a very pragmatic definition stating that 'a survey is a system for collecting information to describe, compare or explain knowledge, attitudes and behaviour. Surveys involve setting objectives for information collection, designing research, preparing a reliable and valid data collection instrument, administering and scoring the instrument, analysing data and reporting the results' (p. 1). Apart from clearly outlining the various stages involved in a survey (and we will return to this later on), Fink explains that surveys can be descriptive, providing answers to straightforward questions such as the composition of a population in terms of gender, marital status, employment history and so on. They can move a step further and investigate people's attitudes and opinions, such as whether they think the range of health-care services available is sufficient and of good quality. Surveys can become more sophisticated by testing hypotheses: for example that mothers with higher levels of education are more likely to breast-feed their children than mothers with lower levels of education. Thus, you need to collect data on mothers with different levels of education and how they feed their babies. Fink warns that you should only include hypothesis testing if you are sure that your research design and the expected data quality justify your doing so.

The surveys that are mostly used by health services researchers can be classified into three types (Mayer, quoted in Baker, 1991).

- **Factual surveys**, which collect and analyse hard, quantitative data on, for example, usage or habits. Questions concerning smoking, physical exercise or dietary intake belong to this type.

- **Opinion surveys,** which focus on people's perceptions of the topics studied. Thus, the type of data collected is subjective and qualitative, often based upon people's own experiences. The study on LLI falls within this category, as do so-called patient satisfaction surveys such as the hospital user feedback study, or asking people's preferences for certain types of treatment.

- **Interpretative surveys** ask people about their beliefs or behaviours and explanations for them. This approach comes closest to the more qualitative types such as the in-depth interview, but by structuring the format more people can be studied. Examples are studies on inequalities in health and testing hypotheses for the persistence of those inequalities (Blaxter, 1997).

Surveys collect a structured set of data. In order to be able to create this structure you must have sufficient background knowledge of the problem or issue to be studied. This basically involves examining the literature in the chosen field, and with the existence of computerized databases and the information available through the Internet, a systematic review of both published and unpublished (so-called grey literature) has been made easier. Surveys carried out in the same subject area are another source of background study and often help you to determine overlaps and gaps in knowledge. Once you are clear about what is already known you can begin to plan the survey.

2.3 WHEN TO USE A SURVEY

The most important question in research design is: What are the objectives of the research? It is through determining the objectives that you decide on methods and the details of the actual research process. Thus, the objectives are a clearly formulated statement of intended outcomes. For example, the Health and Lifestyle Survey (Cox *et al.*, 1987) had as its main objective 'to examine the relationships of lifestyles, behaviours and circumstances to the physical and mental health of a large representative sample of the British population' (Introduction).

Hart (1987) argues that the survey is well suited to delivering the objective of collecting factual, attitudinal and/or behavioural data. Furthermore, it can collect a large amount of information from a wide population in an economical fashion because of its formal nature. The above example of the Health and Lifestyle Survey did precisely that: in order to achieve its objective, data was collected on four major habits – diet, exercise, smoking and alcohol consumption – intending to assess their prevalence and their associations with health and fitness. Furthermore, individuals' beliefs and attitudes to health and health promotion were investigated alongside physiological measures and measures of cognitive functioning, personality and psychiatric status. The scope of the survey was large, covering England, Scotland and Wales and interviewing 9003 individuals.

Fink (1995) warns that the objectives have to be formulated in a precise and unambiguous manner. This is important, as many terms used have multiple meanings depending on the perspective of the person doing or responding to the survey. Thus, in the Health and Lifestyle one of the objectives was to investigate the association between smoking and health. This was done through a number of dimensions, including smoking status. People could classify themselves as 'current regular' or 'current occasional' smokers. The words 'regular' and 'occasional' were relative concepts that could be variously interpreted. They required a precise delineation and 'current regular' was defined as more than one cigarette a day while 'current occasional' was defined as less than one cigarette per day.

Deciding when to do a survey relates to your objectives. In short, you can use a survey when you want to produce descriptive statistics on a whole population, but at a much lower cost than with a census of every member of that population. If you want to map out and measure associations between different factors surveys are appropriate tools. For the study of causal processes, and the developments and testing of explanations for specific associations or social patterns surveys can be employed (Hakim, 1987).

2.4 THE STAGES IN SURVEY DESIGN

Here we will briefly outline the various stages of survey design, which will be elaborated upon in the subsequent chapters. Of course, there are other books that outline these stages in considerable detail and *The Survey Kit* (Fink *et al.*, 1995) is one of the more user-friendly manuals available. Cartwright and Seale (1990) extensively describe the stages of a survey study, including all the problems and difficulties encountered in their research.

The preparation for a survey has already been alluded to when we mentioned literature reviews. Another way to prepare is to consult experts in the field who can assist in sharpening up the objectives for your survey. They can be consulted from a distance (e.g. using postal or electronic mail) or in person. Fink (1995) suggests that setting up meetings with experts in focus groups or consensus panels might be a good way to developing your design and objectives.

The second area for preparation is securing access to the population to be studied. For some studies institutions or individuals operate as a sort of gatekeeper, and they have to be informed of the objectives of the study. Their agreement with the objectives is important if you are to be allowed access to the study population. If individuals are selected through public records such as the electoral roll a direct approach can be made to them. However, if you need to access them through records held by professionals or bodies such as hospitals, permission has to be sought from ethical committees (in the UK context). Cartwright and Seale (1990) have reported their considerable difficulties with ethical committees who need to give approval for research taking place in the health care field that involves people. It is important that you establish whether you require this type of approval and what rules are operating in your local area before you embark upon the research.

In the case of our LLI study we had to gain permission from the local ethical committee because we intended to identify possible respondents through general practice records. Furthermore, we wanted to scrutinize those records in order to compare the clinical assessment with people's self-assessment of their health status. This also meant that we had to design a consent form, which the ethical committee scrutinized.

Another issue concerning access is when the people who can allow access are also the sponsors of the research. Agreement on the objectives of the survey becomes even more important, but on the other hand the question of independence plays a role as well. If sponsors want to influence the objectives – and thus the intended outcomes – of the survey too much you will be confronted with a dilemma concerning scientific integrity and financial support. It is important that scientific standards are not being compromised, which you need to get across in discussions with sponsors. As research takes place in the real world, learning to negotiate is increasingly an essential part of the researcher's role.

Most surveys have a pilot stage, which is designed to test out instruments and iron out problems before they cause major disruption to the main survey. Through what is learned in a pilot the research design can be amended and tools can be changed. Questionnaires often undergo alterations in the wording of questions or the order in which they are asked. Methods of administration can also be piloted and choices can be made between, for example, self-administered questionnaires or interviews. Issues of timing can be sorted out, which was important in the Cartwright and Seale survey (1990), where bereaved relatives were interviewed: if they were interviewed too soon after their bereavement it would be too distressing, if there was a big time gap their memories of the dying process would not necessarily be as clear. Thus, the 'right period' had to be defined with some accuracy.

The pilot areas or individuals included in the pilot study have to be similar to the ones that are part of the main survey in order to allow for valid comparisons. At the same time they cannot be included in the main sample. In our LLI study we piloted in wards that had similar levels of reported LLI to, but fell outside, the GP practice area that was the focus of the survey.

The next stages are covered in detail in Chapters 3 and 4, namely the selection of a sample and questionnaire design. Rigorous sampling methods are the backbone of any survey and the definition of inclusion and exclusion criteria is of crucial importance. We discuss different types of sampling and the vexed question of sample size. The issue of skills and resources does play a role in deciding on sample survey methodology and the extent to which you can try to achieve high response rates.

Fat books have been written about questionnaire design and we will only review the most important issues in Chapter 4. Accuracy, simplicity and lack of ambiguity are key tenets of good questionnaire design. Poor questions will result in poor answers, thus making your data unusable and the questionnaire a waste of time for the respondents and yourself. Furthermore, the reliability and validity of your survey tools require to be tested. This is often done by others if you use 'off-the-shelf' instruments (for a review of health instruments see Bowling, 1994, 1997; Wilkin *et al.*, 1992) or in your pilot study. If you use instruments developed by others you must check whether they are copyright, and a review of studies using the instrument is useful to understand its applicability, and its strengths and weaknesses. If possible, talking to the designers of the tool or previous users to understand potential pitfalls can be useful as well.

Carrying out the main survey is a big task that should be timetabled properly and set against available resources. Using a project management framework can be helpful, especially in planning ahead and determining milestones. Attracting the right staff (if you are so lucky to have the funds) and training them is one consideration, setting up administration systems for tasks such as posting questionnaires, checking responses, sending reminders is another task. Monitoring quality, especially when you are using a large number of interviewers, is important and spot-checks on filled-in questionnaires should be carried out. Maintaining good relationships with a variety of stakeholders should not be forgotten, be they sponsors, gatekeepers or respondents. It is often said that good research depends on the 'social competence' of the researchers and that certainly is the case in our experience. Part of the process is giving feedback to respondents and sponsors, which should not just be done at the end of the study but preferably at key points throughout the study.

If the collection of the data is well organized you should not encounter major difficulties when organizing the data ready for analysis. In Chapter 5 we discuss the ordering of the material and in Chapter 6 we continue methods of summarizing data. In Chapters 7–10 we will discuss the analytical stages. Fink (1995) recommends that you design an analysis plan and remain focused on the objectives defined at the start. It is so easy to get waylaid into all sorts of interesting side-tracks and the analysis plan is meant to keep you on the straight and narrow.

Reporting on the findings is the final and very important stage. An explanation of and justification for the methodology are crucial elements. Not only do you need to demonstrate that you have achieved the objectives of the survey, but in case you did not, to give reasons why. The scientific merit of the survey will largely be judged by the way it is presented and giving due attention to clear and accessible writing is a worthwhile time investment. You want, of course, your reports or articles to be read and wide dissemination is becoming increasingly important, not only for the researcher's own career but also because you and the sponsors want to make an impact in the chosen field. Particularly in the health arena many of the issues researched within surveys have a practical angle and user-friendly reporting makes a big contribution to the survey results being used.

2.5 CONCLUSION

In this chapter we have stressed that the invisible tasks of thinking about survey design and the objectives of the survey are essential to the success of your work. Thus, you must be clear in your own mind what you want to know and how you should be going about finding the answers. You need to be sure about the appropriateness of the design to your research question. From then on the survey takes on a logical structure that has been captured by Fink (1995, pp. 78–80) in the following stages:

- design the survey (sample);
- prepare the survey instrument;
- pilot-test the instrument;
- administer the instrument;
- organize the data;
- analyse the data;
- report the results.

3 SAMPLE SURVEYS

3.1 INTRODUCTION

The idea behind sample surveys is to collect information about a population and to draw inferences about that **population** based on collecting the information about only part of that population, known as the **sample**. For example, in our limiting long-term illness (LLI) project, the population is everyone aged 18 and over registered at one general practice and our sample is 4044 patients we have selected, randomly, to ask questions of to represent this population

Imagine a database containing records of patients registered at a particular general practice. Each record will identify one particular patient and will contain different information relating to each patient. Although each patient will have information under the same headings (e.g. age, sex, postcode, date of last consultation, active problems and medication) it would be most unlikely to have two or more patients with identical records. These individual characteristics of the record will vary among patients and, hence, are known as **variables**. We are likely to want to measure values of different variables from the sample and to test these against prior hypotheses about the population. All surveys should have a main aim and any secondary aims, which are stated before discussion of the methodology needed is started. Related to these will be particular variables that need to be measured.

A characteristic that will be the same for all patients is that they are all registered at the same general practice; hence, this is known as a **constant**. The constants will further describe the particular population to which the results of the survey are applicable. Hence, a sample survey of general practice patients will be applicable to the general practice population.

In the limiting long-term illness project described in Chapters 1 and 2, the main variable under consideration in stage 1 is the self reporting of an LLI or not; a simple Yes–No variable. Here, only the 1991 Census question asking a person whether they had an illness, handicap or disability that limited their normal daily activities (described normally as a limiting long-term illness) was sent to respondents. The second stage is slightly more complicated in that the questionnaire used was the Short Form-36 (SF-36), which is described in Appendix C. This has eight different health scales, measuring dimensions of health such as general health, physical functioning and mental health, with scores for each person on each scale ranging from 0 (worst health) to 100 (best health). The main scale chosen was General Health, as it allows people to give their own general opinions on their health (while not forgetting the importance and rich stream of information we can glean from the other scales). In this stage, a second survey was performed using the SF-36 to allow us to compare results on the SF-36 between people who reported an LLI in stage 1 and a sample of people who said they had no LLI.

In the patient satisfaction survey set in a hospital, the main characteristic measured (which was set within a questionnaire) was satisfaction with a preassessment visit before going into hospital.

Other examples of variables we might wish to collect information on might be the number of units of alcohol drunk in a week by teenagers, the job satisfaction of nurses at a general hospital or the length of distance needed to travel to attend an outpatients clinic. These examples all relate to human beings, but while the subject of enquiry often is people it need not always be so. For example, we may wish to investigate the quality of food at hospitals, the number of baked beans in similar-sized tins of different brands or the speed over 5 metres of tortoises. However, much of what follows will assume measurement on individuals. Obviously, you are likely to want to ask many different questions, as in the second stage of the LLI survey, but there should be one main question you want answered.

Now, stop! Before proceeding with a survey the first thing you need to do is to consider a checklist of actions, described in Table 3.1.

Table 3.1	
Issues in survey design	• Define **purpose** of survey • Determine study population of interest • Determine sample frame • Decide method of collection of data • Decide on type of survey • Determine sample size • Start thinking of **analysis** of resultant data

The second thing is to go and seek advice from a statistician, or at least someone experienced in research design. S/he will be able to advise and keep you on the right track. Having said that, for a research project (that is your baby) you will need to have enough knowledge to formulate your own research methodology and just require the odd bit of specialist advice or agreement at certain stages. Please carry on and we will consider the actions in Table 3.1 in turn.

There are a number of different designs for collecting quantitative information, of which this text deals with two of the most common. Experiments, in which the experimenter has control over the units, are one form. For example, a study of sleep deprivation where the experimenter may control the number of hours of sleep a person has and discover how this affects his/her performance in simple tests is one form of experiment. A particular form of experiment called randomized control trials will be covered in Chapter 11.

Sample surveys is obviously a big area, and many texts have been written on the subject. In this chapter it is only possible to cover the basics and to get your mind on the right track. Possible further reading on sample survey design includes Barnett, 1991, Fowler, 1993 and Moser and Kalton, 1971.

3.2 WHAT IS A SAMPLE SURVEY?

The idea behind sample surveys is to collect information as efficiently and effectively as possible. Instead of asking questions of everyone registered at our general practice we intended to ask only a proportion of the patients. In effect, therefore, we will elicit information from a number of individuals (known as the **sample**) to find out more about the population from which we have extracted them. By collecting and analysing data from only part of a population, we wish to be able to make conclusions with confidence about the population as a whole. Next time you are in a restaurant and you reach over and try a little bit of your dinner companion's food you are, in fact, sampling his/her food!

It is at this point that readers should remember the famous saying that 'Statistics is never having to say you are certain' but, in this respect, statistics is like life itself. There are few things you can rely on in life. However, this does not mean we should give up hope. Any competent survey reported in a competent journal will give details on the type of survey used, sample size and method of sampling and each of these components can help to reduce the error and bias that could infect a survey. To get results from the sample that reflect the population as accurately as possible, we need to eliminate this error and bias by as much as possible. For example, we would not expect a health profile of people aged 85 and over to accurately represent the health of the whole population.

3.3 WHY PERFORM A SAMPLE SURVEY?

3.3.1 Is there a need?

To some people surveying is instinctive. Give them a research problem and, immediately, it is out with the questionnaires, get those interview techniques sharpened up and let us see if we can get more responses than old Muggins over there got on his survey of the medicine taken by deep-sea fishermen with hayfever. However, to perform a survey when it is unnecessary or has no chance of obtaining reliable results is uneconomic and unethical if those results are published as fact when they are known to be highly inaccurate.

The first reaction should be to attempt to discover whether the information required is available already, whether in previous surveys asking the same question and with the same conditions (e.g. the population from which the sample is drawn should be similar, with the same background characteristics) or through records such as medical records or other sources like national Census data. A trawl through the relevant literature is important as the first stage, to see if similar surveys have been performed (possibly making this one redundant), as a basis for searching for possible questionnaires (which will be discussed in the next chapter), for understanding the population you want information about and the subject involved and, at least if a similar survey is revealed, as a means of comparing data from your survey. Analysis of the 1991 UK Census data allowed us to obtain background socioeconomic features of the area of our LLI study and compare our prevalence rates for LLI (percentage of respondents with an LLI) with those obtained in the Census.

A second question must be whether our intended respondents have the information we require and also whether they are willing and able (legally and morally) to share that information with us. Questions of a highly personal nature (such as sexual habits) may obtain no or 'false' (i.e. incorrect) answers. In the UK, questions on income are often regarded as taboo. While many countries, such as Australia and the USA, include questions on income in their national censuses, Great Britain currently does not. Piloting of questions in this case is all-important and will be discussed in the next chapter.

3.3.2 Why not perform a complete census?

If sample surveys are prone to error and bias then the question might arise as to why not simply perform a complete census. There are a number of reasons why a sample survey is a better option than a complete census. It is often impossible to ask questions of everybody in a population (which may be a million or more). Not all errors that result are necessarily a result of sampling rather than performing a complete census (what are called sampling errors), as will be seen later. However, it would be unwise to sample when a census would be just as practical and plausible.

The first main reason is, obviously, cost. Surveys should be cheaper to perform. We are, after all, obtaining information from fewer people. Unfortunately, we are normally constrained by limited time and resources. Secondly, there is the problem of accessibility. Some people may be difficult to access or identify (could you produce a list of drug dealers in your area? If so, contact the police!). Thirdly, speed: sample surveys will be quicker than censuses. The amount of fieldwork is obviously reduced, as will be the data recording and entry. This is vital if the data is needed urgently. Finally, and perhaps surprisingly, there is the question of accuracy. It is a nice characteristic of surveys that, often, accurate results can be obtained from a sample consisting of just a small proportion of a population. Errors can be reduced by careful consideration of a sample survey design and efficient use of skilled workforce, rather than a hurried census, using a larger, less skilled workforce. Often the only point of a census is to obtain precise information about subdivisions; with these subdivisions being too small or too numerous to allow sampling from them. The 10-yearly national Census can supply information on ethnic groups, for example, for different age groups, in different localities and with different socioeconomic backgrounds. A national sample survey of the whole UK population would be unlikely to obtain enough people from all these subdivisions to obtain this information accurately for each and every subdivision. Sampling from each of the subdivisions would also be time-consuming and complicated, and the sample size needed may make it just as worthwhile to survey everyone. A final reason is that the sample process can often destroy the units involved. Your dinner companion might not be too impressed if, in trying their food, you ate all of it!

3.4 INITIAL CONSIDERATIONS

The most important part of a survey is to ask yourself: What is the main aim of this survey? There are likely to be many sub-aims but you should constantly remind yourself of the primary aim and concentrate on that. In our LLI survey, the main aim in the first stage was to obtain the prevalence of LLI in the patients registered at the practice and, in the second stage, to compare the LLI group with the non-LLI group on the scores from the SF-36; particularly on General Health. Other comparisons, such as comparing scores between those who had consulted their GP in the past 3 months and those who had not, or considering demographic details from the demographic questionnaire of those with different conditions extracted from their medical records, were considered secondary. Another question is: Which factors do we feel will influence our results? These could be age, sex, type of illness or social class, for example. These will either have to be obtained during the survey or, if known beforehand, controlled for in the research design. That is why we included a demographic questionnaire alongside the SF-36 in our survey.

The next question is to decide how wide or narrow to make our **study population** (i.e. the population from which the sample will be drawn). We begin with a **target population**; this is the population we want information about. This is often quite general. For example, in our LLI study, our target population is the patients registered with the general practice. However, because of the practicalities of performing a survey, it is normal to strictly define a study population based on certain inclusion criteria and exclusion criteria. In our LLI study, we would have problems dealing with people who left the practice after the start of the survey but before analysis started, and with those who joined after the start date. The decision, therefore, was that the sample would be selected from everybody registered with the practice on the date we regarded as the 'official' start of the survey (the **inclusion criteria**) as joiners and leavers were expected to be few over the lifetime of the project. Secondly, age was a concern. Our study was concentrating on adults and not on the special problems of children. Therefore, an **exclusion criteria** was: everybody under 18 years of age registered at the practice on the 'official' start date.

What must be remembered is that data obtained can only be related to the study population; in other words, in our LLI project our data relates to those aged 18 and over registered with the practice at the time of the start of the project. **Eligibility criteria** must be constructed and kept to rigidly. For example, consider a survey on smokers, the target population being simply defined as 'smokers'. Decisions must be made as to whether the research is to concentrate on all smokers (including 'occasion' such as birthday and Christmas smokers), just regular smokers (at least one a day) or heavy smokers (10 or more a day, for example). Also, does this include cigar smokers or just cigarette smokers? Underage smokers? We need to develop inclusion and exclusion criteria from which to define our study population. Whatever you decide now will influence your results and conclusions. Each person who fits your criteria will become a member of the study population, nominally a **sampling unit**, and should have an equal chance of being selected for the study. As stated before, we have used people as our example but it could equally be hospitals or addresses.

Once we have defined our study population, we still have a problem. We need a **sample frame**, which is simply a list of all the sampling units. It could be a piece of paper or a computer database but should be identical to the study population. Each sampling unit should be included once, and once only, on the sampling frame. The LLI sample frame was simply the general practice register filtered by exclusion criteria. A study of health needs assessment of the elderly used a sample frame taken from the local Family Health Services Authority – FHSA – (as it then was) register excluding those aged under 65 years at the start date of the study. Other potential frames include electoral registers, computerized lists of patients in hospitals and computerized payrolls.

Problems in sample frames include incomplete frames or people on the frame who have died or moved who should have been removed from it. These problems may either mean adjustment of the study population definition or may induce bias into our results if there are people who fit the criteria of our study population but have no chance of being selected because they are not on the frame or, alternatively, there are people on the frame who should not be. If we were to do a survey of a particular geographical district but used the telephone book as our frame we would be omitting not only those who are ex-directory but also those without a phone (normally the poorer end of the population), hence incorporating an obvious bias into our survey.

Other problems involving sample frames include actually getting hold of one. The problem of obtaining a sample frame for drug dealers has already been raised and problems involving general population sample frames can arise in many areas of the world. The section dealing with types of sampling will consider ways around a faulty (or completely absent) sample frame.

3.5 METHODS OF OBTAINING DATA

There are a number of methods of obtaining data but the two most common are through **face-to-face interviews** and by **postal surveys**. First of all, though, we will have a quick look at two other methods of obtaining data in sample surveys before investigating the pros and cons of the two most common methods.

3.5.1 Recorded or published information

Recorded information or published studies can be sampled or analysed as a whole. This includes data like national Census data, medical records and previous surveys from the literature. A special case of producing quantitative reviews of a subject (e.g. the relationship between type of occupation and the prevalence of asthma, or whether smoking during pregnancy is related to low birth weight) based on research of the literature and studies performed and published by others is called a **meta-analysis**. Meta-analysis essentially involves finding all the studies that have been performed on a particular subject, e.g. the effect of a particular treatment for a disease, and combining all the data together by statistical analysis. The advantages of this is that it allows us to assess the evidence from a number of studies in the same area at the same time and it overcomes the problems of individual studies being too small to detect any real statistical significance. Two of the problems of meta-analysis (although a common procedure) that need to be overcome are that, firstly, the research studies published in the literature are all likely to have different characteristics, such as being based on different populations, using different types of analysis or using different methods of sampling; although it may well be that we can obtain a wider generalization of the results by combining studies with slightly different populations. Secondly, there is a possible bias in the literature whereby studies with significant results are more likely to get published. For example, studies showing that a particular method of surgery is more effective than another method may be more inclined to be accepted for publication than studies showing no difference in the effectiveness of the two methods (for more on the problems and features of publication bias see Begg and Berlin, 1988; Easterbrook *et al.*, 1991). For more on meta-analysis see, for example, Petitti, 1994 or Chapter 17 in Bland, 1995.

A thorough review of randomized controlled trials in a particular area without the statistical analysis is called a **systematic review** (see Chambers and Altman, 1995 for more details).

The main problem with recorded information is that it is usually produced for a different purpose from that for which you require it. Therefore, such data can only act as pointers. They are also often going to be out of date and often too aggregated for your particular uses. The national Census, for example, is collected every 10 years and the full Census data set is available at enumeration district level at its lowest level, although it is possible to sample anonymized individual records. Secondary data is often best used as background information, either as a starting point for research or as an indicator of what should be investigated. The LLI project began by studying the national Census data, which revealed that the district of Stoke-on-Trent had the eighth highest rate of limiting long-term illness out of the 366 districts in England when standardized by age and sex (i.e. calculating LLI rates for each district based on the age and sex distribution for England as a whole so that comparisons can be made on LLI without the influence of different age and sex distributions – Forrest and Gordon, 1995) and had the sixth highest ratio of people with limiting long-term illness to health care professionals, with 215 people with an LLI to every health care professional (Gordon and Forrest, 1995). This revealed the particular importance of limiting long-term illness in the Stoke area.

3.5.2 Telephone

An increasingly common method of obtaining data, particularly common in market research and in selling, is by using the telephone. A major advantage of telephone interviewing is that it is less time-consuming and requires fewer interviewers than face-to-face interviews. It is becoming more and more popular. However, the major problem of this method is that it immediately introduces a bias. Only people who actually have a telephone can, obviously, be sampled. As people without telephones are likely to be from the poorer end of the income spectrum (and from the lower end of the social class), then there can be a major skew in the results. Obviously, this depends on the population targeted. In some populations, e.g. businesses in the UK, all potential units will have a telephone (however, some might have more than one phone number, which would need to be recognized if, in some form, the numbers are 'picked out of a hat'). However, elsewhere, in poorer sections of the community, it may be the case that only 50% of the target population has a telephone. Another problem arises if selections are made by using the telephone directory, because this immediately rules out people with ex-directory numbers.

Aside from the sample selection problems, telephone interviewing may increase response errors with concentration problems; you cannot be sure, for example, whether people are concentrating half on the questions on the phone and half on their favourite television programme! There may be problems with mishearing or misunderstanding of questions over the telephone and of feelings of intrusion by the anticipated respondent, reducing the response rate and increasing the chance of a false answer. There will also be problems in using telephone surveys with people with hearing problems.

A number of the pros and cons ascribed to face-to-face interviews below also relate to telephone interviews. Telephones are often, and perhaps most successfully, used as a means of following up non-respondents from a postal survey. For more on telephone survey methodology for a nursing study see Barriball *et al.*, 1996 and for general practitioner surveys in a comparison with a postal survey, Sibbald *et al.*, 1994.

3.5.3 Postal or face-to-face?

Table 3.2 gives a concise check of the advantages and disadvantages of postal surveys as opposed to face-to-face interviews. Both methods have their pros and cons and are favoured by different types of people for different occasions.

Postal surveys have the main advantage of being less costly. The questionnaires can be sent out and returned (using a stamped addressed return envelope supplied with the questionnaire or a business reply-paid envelope) for the cost of two (second class) stamps. In face-to-face

Advantages	Disadvantages	Table 3.2
• Less time consuming • Less expensive (normally) • No interviewer bias • Wider geographical coverage • Completed at respondent's convenience	• Smaller response rate • Totally structured • At least one reminder (sometimes more) usually required • Needs longer period of time • Problems of illiteracy • Problems of poor postal service	The pros and cons of using a postal survey as opposed to a face-to-face survey

interviews, the interviewers have to be paid and their expenses also met. While the mundane work of filling envelopes will need to be done, it is unlikely to match the cost of interviewers. It also allows a wider geographical coverage without large increases in cost and necessitates less manpower to sample the same number, usually allowing larger numbers to be sampled in a postal survey. Postal surveys will also be less time-consuming. After the initial effort of filling envelopes, it is simply a matter of sitting back and waiting for the questionnaires to return, unlike face-to-face interviews where the interviews themselves, and travelling to and from the place of interview, will consume time. However, while these interviews, with a reasonable number of interviewers, may be able to be performed over a short period of time, postal surveys can stretch over a number of months. There is likely to be the need for at least one reminder to people who have not replied to the original questionnaire. This may be in the form of a postcard reminding the potential respondent about the survey, or another questionnaire. Further reminders may be necessary; and if a postcard has been sent for the first reminder than subsequent reminders should be another copy of the questionnaire.

Postal surveys have been shown to obtain lower **response rates** than face-to-face interviews. Response rates are the percentage of the selected sample who complete questionnaires or agree to, and have, face-to-face interviews. Possible methods of increasing response rates will be described in section 3.8 and good questionnaire design is very important and will be covered in the next chapter. The lower the response rate, the more chance there is of obtaining 'false' results. If the non-respondents have particular characteristics that would lead to them giving different answers from the norm for the respondents, then the survey team are in trouble. Often a figure of around 40–45% response for each administration of the questionnaire is quoted as 'typical' for postal surveys (i.e. 40% response rate for the original survey, 40% response from the remaining 60% sent first reminders, 40% response from the remaining 36% of the original sample sent second reminders and so on). The actual response rate will depend on the type of population surveyed and the questions asked. Further discussion about the response rate will be made later.

Questionnaire design is very important whether postal, face-to-face or telephone surveys are used, but is particularly important for postal surveys where it will be the only point of contact between the research team and the respondent. Postal surveys, therefore, will have to be totally structured, with the questions asked limited to those on the questionnaire, and need to be clear, unbiased, unambiguous and in a form that can be self-completed. Questionnaire design is considered in the next chapter. Face-to-face interviews can be totally structured, with the interviewer simply reading the questions from the questionnaire; semi-structured, which allows the interviewer to follow up questions on the questionnaire allowing for more information; or unstructured, which may mean just a checklist of points to cover allowing the respondent a substantial amount of licence to guide the interview content. In this respect, the face-to-face interviews provides much more scope to select the amount of structure needed and what is best suited for the purpose to hand. Problems concern correct and vigorous training of interviewers to maintain unbiased and consistent interviewing and correct recording of answers. Even inflections in certain parts of a question can change the meaning of a question or imply that a certain answer is expected.

Postal questionnaires have the advantage that they can be answered at the respondent's convenience and without the pressure s/he may feel in the unnatural setting of an interview. However, before setting out on postal surveys information should be sought on levels of illiteracy, different languages spoken (similarly for face-to-face interviews, as for needing questionnaires translated into different languages, it may be necessary to find interviewers capable of speaking different languages) and the quality of the postal service. Some developing countries have poor, or virtually non-existent, postal services. Similarly, it may not be such a good idea to conduct a postal survey in the midst of a postal strike.

3.5.4 The case of the LLI

A number of factors determined the use of a postal survey for the LLI study. These were:

- the main questionnaire used, the Short Form-36, had previously been tested and validated for use in a postal survey. It had been used effectively by this research team in a postal setting in a previous study and can be completed in under 10 minutes. An interesting comparison in the use of the SF-36 in a postal and a telephone setting is given in McHorney *et al.* (1994), who found that respondents from the postal survey had a higher response rate but tended to have worse health. The telephone survey was also much more expensive.

- use of a postal survey meant a higher number of people could be surveyed and thus increased the power and statistical viability of the survey (see section 3.7 for guidance on sample size). The required size of the survey and the smallness of the research team also meant that the use of face-to-face interviews was never going to be practically possible. There was no great enthusiasm for performing face-to-face interviews with 4000 people! Time, while a factor, was not strictly limited, meaning that a speedy, small face-to-face survey was not required.

- study of the Census data revealed that 98% of the population of the area were white UK/European so the use of different languages was not considered necessary and there were no indications that there was a high level of illiteracy.

In contrast, the hospital preassessment visit satisfaction survey was performed face-to-face. The sample size (only 50), the fact that it was a pilot study and that we wanted to encourage comments in addition to the structured questionnaire meant that face-to-face interviews was the most favourable option. Neither interviewer was involved in the actual preassessment and both were trained in interviewing beforehand.

The method of obtaining information is, therefore, very much down to the particular characteristics of your study. Background reading on previous, similar surveys, uses of the questionnaire if used before and understanding the characteristics of the study population is required. You need to choose a form that will obtain the most accurate answers while remaining within your resource constraints. Fowler (1993) gives more discussion of the various methods of data collection.

3.6 TYPES OF SAMPLING

We still have a long way to go in our quest for a solid sample survey design. Remember, a reputable journal or report will necessitate justification of methods used. Remember also that what we are trying to do is to reduce the amount of bias and error in our survey. One key way of doing this is through selection of a judicious type of sampling. How do you actually select people from your sample frame to be in your sample? Often when talking to people conducting surveys about how they selected from their study population they will say that they just took a random sample. In fact, pure, simple random samples are reasonably rare and what they really did was take some type of convenience sample. Maybe it had some form of randomness to it, but most probably it was selected from the people most convenient to sample. Whether the data they ended up with can be related back with any degree of accuracy to their 'believed' study population is, often, debatable.

It is important to know what claims you can, and cannot, make about your results. If we wished to perform a health profile survey for patients registered with a general practice and decided to select every patient who came through the surgery's doors over a period of 1 month, it would be ill-advised for us to suggest that the results reflected the health of the practice population, as a whole, as we have only been measuring the health of those actually attending the surgery over this period. This cohort is, by virtue of having actually visited the surgery, more likely to have ill-health than the practice population as a whole.

The first three types of sampling, which we will only briefly discuss – i.e. **accessibility, judgemental** and **quota** – are all prone to error and bias. They are forms of non-probability sampling. However, we mention them as we promised to suggest ways of overcoming an inadequate or absent sample frame. All these methods are ways around a lack of a sample frame, although their failings should be kept in mind. Another advantage of these methods is that they can be useful as a basis for trying out questionnaires and piloting your survey (see Chapter 4 for a description of pilot surveys and the necessity of doing them). However, generally we would avoid them.

The other types all can reduce error and bias in surveys and improve the results in terms of accuracy and content of information **if used in the right way at the right time.** Again, it will be a matter of generally describing the types, giving examples of their use, without an extensive, in-depth look at them. See the suggested further reading for more detail. Table 3.3 gives a brief summary of the different types of sampling.

Table 3.3		
Types of sampling	**Non-probability**	
	Accessibility	Selecting most convenient units
	Judgemental	Deliberately drawing the sample based on belief of what is most representative of the population as a whole
	Quota	Filling quotas of judgemental different groups of the population by accessibility sampling
	Probability	
	Simple random	Every unit in the study population has an equal chance of being selected
	Systematic	Selecting every kth unit on the sample frame
	Stratified	Dividing study population into heterogeneous subpopulations and sampling from each
	Cluster	Dividing study population into homogeneous subpopulations and selecting one or more of these clusters as representative of population

3.6.1 Accessibility sampling

This is a method of sampling by selecting units most convenient for you. An example of this is randomly visiting houses during working hours or arranging to perform interviews with people who are available during these working hours. This will normally mean that your sample is mainly made up of housewives (or househusbands), the unemployed and shift workers (who probably will not be best pleased at being woken up, and this is a good time to remind you that respondents have to want to answer your questions) and eliminate those who work during the day. This may be effective if these are the people you want to survey but there are still more effective and efficient ways of doing this.

3.6.2 Judgemental sampling

This method involves the experimenter deliberately drawing the sample based on what he or she believes is most representative of the population as a whole. For example, s/he may believe that the elderly makes up a certain percentage of the population and so s/he will try to get this proportion of over-65-year-olds in the sample. In doing so, the experimenter tries to eliminate anticipated sources of distortion and, while this may work up to a point, problems may arise through lack of knowledge or personal prejudices leading to (for the experimenter) unanticipated sources of distortion. If, for example, the experimenter underestimates the number of elderly people in a population, then this section of the community will be under-represented in his/her survey.

3.6.3 Quota sampling

This is a common method of sampling, particularly in market research. The reason why the market researcher will choose you as you scurry past in a desperate dash to get by without being caught, while ignoring others who leisurely stroll by, is that she has a quota of different types of people (maybe based on age, sex, ethnicity or occupational class) that she has been told to fill and, unluckily, you fall into one of those categories. Quota sampling can be looked upon as a combination of accessibility and judgement sampling and may be the only practical solution if there is no sample frame. It can be time-consuming to fill the quotas and needs well-trained interviewers both in selecting people and in asking the questions and recording the answers. However, there is always the possibility of not correctly filling the quotas. Imagine a market researcher interested in selecting professional people for a survey. She may ignore the paint-splashed, overall-wearing consultant nipping out to buy a tin of paint while in the midst of decorating his spare bedroom and pick on a long-term unemployed man wearing a suit for the first time in 2 years as he needs to impress the benefits office. The difficulties involved in judgemental sampling also abound in selecting the type and size of the quotas.

3.6.4 Simple random sampling

Simple random sampling, or SRS, can be defined very simply as selecting the sampling units such that every unit in the study population has an equal chance of being selected. This is the first of the probability sampling methods that we have come across in that each member of the study population has an equal probability of being selected. It is, if you like, the purest form of sampling and relies on a perfect sampling frame; i.e. comprehensive and no repeated units. It is the basis for the other probability-type sampling methods.

There are various methods of actually performing the selection of a SRS. The easiest is to consecutively number the units (e.g. people) on the sampling frame and then use either a computer program that will give a list of random numbers (common in most computer spreadsheet or statistical packages), or randomized numbers tables, which can be found in most sample survey texts. Using these tables will also give you a list of randomized numbers and the units corresponding to these numbers can be selected. Tables 3.4 and 3.5 give abstracts of random numbers tables that we have generated using the random number generator in commercially available software. We cannot testify as to how completely random these tables are!

Suppose we wished to sample from a population numbering 300. We would pick any point in the random numbers table (such as Table 3.4) and start reading across in threes and select the corresponding numbered units in the population. It is wise to start at a different point for each different use of the table. We would also be able to work in multiples of three; for example, unit 1 would be selected if we read 001, 301 or 601, unit 2 if we read 002, 302 or 602, etc. We would ignore the number 000 and numbers from 901 to 999. So, let us use the start of line 10 from Table 3.4 as our basis for selecting our (imaginary) sample.

35905 48890 76764 96444 06574 79907 42799 53415

Then reduce this to sets of three figures:

359 054 889 076 764 964 440 657 479 907 427 995 341

The first group of three is 359. This is higher than 300 so we take 300 away from it and we are left with 59. Our first selection is the unit (i.e. the person) numbered 59. The next group of three is 054 so the person numbered 54 is chosen. This continues as below.

We would select:

- unit 59 (359 – 300)
- unit 54
- unit 289 (889 – 600)
- unit 76
- unit 164 (764 – 600)
- ignore 964
- unit 140 (440 – 300)

and so on moving across and down the random numbers table until we had selected our required size of sample.

As you can see, each unit has an equal chance of being drawn. If, for example, '059' or '659' had been read as well as '359' we would ignore it as we are **sampling without replacement,** i.e. units can only be picked once. If we were **sampling with replacement**, then units could be selected more than once. If we had allowed the numbers 901–999 to have been chosen, then units 1 to 99 would have had a greater chance of being selected than the rest (4/1000 rather than 3/1000).

If you look closely you will see that Table 3.5 is slightly different

Line							
1	31588	90481	20012	02535	33944	39892	90789	43737
2	01034	53902	09127	68701	76145	75196	57821	81077
3	99955	64107	67518	32233	38629	07452	28767	96793
4	85842	82773	30925	49889	57418	30776	62778	06905
5	99559	42848	69410	05645	69510	58026	43432	75865
6	55415	57275	58901	78101	56116	52511	89245	97959
7	21880	84102	68445	38397	71892	30985	06781	82209
8	19130	95689	41288	60042	28244	90141	00736	08031
9	45932	27908	92527	55137	48178	16058	85276	71795
10	35905	48890	76764	96444	06574	79907	42799	53415
11	37168	16784	53694	11792	28569	22830	80301	75095
12	94450	29532	18994	14338	36750	57400	26294	88301
13	56802	55449	70331	45184	72619	71930	36274	70195
14	81144	88368	22360	89505	95886	23967	10488	32617
15	09928	78183	80193	37305	88369	65264	99059	85884
16	21101	78310	33828	68876	46274	21965	81546	93978
17	99894	59251	49652	02084	88877	64324	94929	16619
18	71003	01023	87441	98291	79624	70163	15703	26435
19	11390	46690	61671	42166	46691	60481	32384	93174
20	40222	04824	48490	52496	31328	23528	54415	41278
21	31588	90481	20012	02353	33944	39892	90789	43737
22	01034	53902	09127	68701	76145	75196	57821	81077
23	99955	64107	67518	32233	38629	07452	28767	96793
24	85842	82773	30925	49889	57418	30776	62778	06905
25	99559	42848	69410	05645	69510	58026	43432	75865
26	55415	57275	58901	78101	56116	52511	89245	97959
27	21880	84102	68445	38397	71892	30985	06781	82209
28	19130	95689	41288	60042	28244	90141	00736	08031
29	45932	27908	92527	55137	48178	16058	85276	71795
30	35905	48890	76764	96444	06574	79907	42799	53415
31	37168	16784	53694	11792	28569	22830	80301	75095
32	94450	29532	18984	14338	36750	57400	26294	88301
33	56802	55449	70331	45184	72619	71930	36274	70195
34	81144	88368	22360	89505	95886	23967	10488	32617
35	09928	78183	80193	37305	88369	65264	99059	85884
36	21101	77831	03382	86887	64627	42196	58154	69397
37	99894	59251	49652	02084	88877	64324	94929	16619
38	71003	01023	87441	98291	79624	70163	15703	26435
39	11390	46690	61671	42166	46691	60481	32384	93174
40	40222	04824	48490	52496	31328	23528	54415	41278
41	76180	70896	86008	86312	12619	74326	80034	94512
42	09519	09012	28391	36077	99351	40042	21380	74331
43	90778	78197	32599	78062	77750	41012	27149	25874
44	24129	52684	22915	93585	92398	62982	71400	11815
45	39570	61816	04009	27795	53085	52340	20514	63676
46	27819	47621	45373	39150	56524	68248	68151	73413
47	93186	81829	02216	77451	18130	40332	80624	47612
48	57808	16494	77567	71668	20395	38040	74780	46716
49	29221	15167	11626	50093	91916	37157	30811	85543
50	70514	59770	12411	08105	49846	46274	53724	77399

Table 3.4

Example of a random numbers table

3 Sample surveys

Table 3.5

Example of a random numbers table; numbers 0 to 19 randomly ordered

Line																				
1	16	17	5	14	9	18	10	12	8	11	6	2	3	19	1	15	4	7	0	13
2	4	19	14	18	16	0	2	13	1	12	17	6	3	5	10	7	15	8	9	11
3	8	3	12	1	11	10	18	5	13	15	0	2	14	17	9	6	4	7	16	19
4	18	2	3	8	10	6	11	17	19	14	13	4	5	12	0	16	15	7	1	9
5	1	5	10	7	19	3	18	12	14	1	4	17	9	13	6	2	8	0	11	15
6	0	14	2	17	6	15	12	10	9	4	7	1	3	16	11	18	13	5	19	8
7	6	0	14	13	1	7	19	3	9	8	16	2	10	12	17	5	18	4	15	11
8	14	10	7	18	12	16	3	17	11	9	1	4	0	15	2	8	5	19	6	13
9	0	9	19	6	13	16	2	1	11	3	15	8	10	18	17	7	5	14	12	4
10	8	2	14	15	0	17	18	10	19	7	11	6	9	16	3	13	12	5	4	1
11	4	5	19	8	6	2	14	3	16	18	12	11	7	10	0	13	9	1	15	17
12	16	19	0	13	17	8	11	6	4	2	1	10	14	7	9	3	18	5	12	15
13	16	8	19	11	4	17	15	14	18	1	10	3	2	13	9	6	0	7	12	5
14	3	14	10	0	12	17	11	1	2	6	18	15	8	7	5	19	4	16	9	13
15	7	1	9	10	16	4	15	19	0	18	2	3	5	6	8	17	12	13	11	14
16	8	3	17	9	15	10	1	18	2	16	0	13	11	19	14	4	12	6	7	5
17	5	6	8	1	12	11	2	4	14	13	10	19	7	3	16	17	15	0	9	18
18	13	12	7	9	5	17	11	1	0	15	2	18	6	14	8	19	3	4	10	16
19	19	1	7	4	3	9	2	11	13	5	10	15	12	17	6	14	18	16	0	8
20	19	0	6	12	18	8	3	9	13	14	17	5	1	15	7	2	11	4	10	16
21	17	13	15	16	9	19	4	1	3	0	14	18	2	5	12	10	6	8	11	7
22	5	6	17	16	19	1	13	8	0	14	3	12	15	9	18	11	7	10	2	4
23	9	18	14	5	10	15	0	19	8	1	11	13	2	12	16	6	3	17	7	4
24	3	1	9	12	13	5	16	7	14	0	2	15	6	18	11	8	4	10	19	17
25	11	13	16	19	17	3	1	18	12	0	14	5	9	10	4	2	8	6	15	7
26	18	7	12	9	15	0	19	17	3	8	11	5	1	14	13	10	6	16	4	2
27	11	1	2	9	6	14	15	19	17	12	7	3	10	5	0	8	18	13	16	4
28	12	7	19	16	9	4	3	15	14	18	8	11	17	1	6	5	10	2	13	0
29	11	0	1	19	8	14	3	6	18	4	17	16	5	10	9	13	7	2	15	12
30	6	8	7	2	1	10	11	17	18	0	4	5	9	15	3	16	19	12	14	13
31	7	8	3	12	10	4	5	14	0	1	11	2	18	13	15	16	9	6	17	19
32	1	3	2	7	9	15	5	14	17	18	16	8	12	11	13	10	19	6	4	0
33	18	6	8	7	10	3	0	2	19	17	1	11	16	9	14	13	15	4	12	5
34	0	13	7	5	17	11	18	8	15	16	3	10	4	19	14	1	12	6	9	2
35	10	15	2	3	13	19	12	18	1	9	7	16	6	11	0	5	17	4	14	8
36	4	16	9	14	17	6	7	18	5	15	1	11	0	13	19	2	8	12	10	3
37	15	10	1	4	3	16	18	0	8	5	6	12	17	2	13	9	14	11	19	7
38	0	11	14	15	17	1	10	7	18	16	2	12	9	4	6	13	5	8	19	3
39	11	8	2	13	5	10	14	4	18	17	12	7	9	3	16	6	0	15	1	19
40	12	9	1	17	2	16	10	7	19	3	4	0	13	15	5	18	8	11	6	14
41	10	0	13	17	16	6	14	4	5	12	19	15	8	1	18	11	2	7	3	9
42	12	10	13	3	2	19	16	1	4	5	18	6	11	9	14	0	8	15	17	7
43	3	17	8	11	14	12	4	1	9	5	19	16	6	0	13	10	18	7	2	15
44	1	4	0	2	7	17	16	9	19	3	12	5	10	14	15	13	6	11	8	18
45	17	8	2	6	5	10	13	9	11	0	4	16	1	12	15	19	7	14	3	18
46	10	5	19	11	9	14	0	13	8	15	16	6	18	1	17	2	4	12	7	3
47	16	15	10	3	11	13	9	7	17	18	18	12	2	8	14	1	4	0	5	6
48	15	0	19	2	12	9	7	14	17	1	6	4	3	13	5	16	10	18	11	8
49	13	16	3	18	11	4	1	5	12	2	8	17	9	10	14	15	7	19	6	0
50	19	6	9	1	2	16	10	15	4	0	8	12	18	5	11	17	14	7	3	13

from Table 3.4 in that each number from 0–19 is included once, and only once, in each row. This is useful if you wanted to arrange in order 20 or fewer units or select from a study population of 20 or less. Also, say we wanted to test the effectiveness of three drugs for hayfever, then we could allocate drug 1 the numbers 1, 4, 7, 10, 13 and 16; drug 2 the numbers 2, 5, 8, 11, 14 and 17 and drug 3 the numbers 3, 6, 9, 12, 15 and 18. Then for each successive patient we could read the next number in our selected row and allocate them the drug matching that number to that patient. See Pocock, 1983, Chapter 5 for more on selecting from random numbers tables.

The National Lottery in the UK is an example of a simple random sample where each number from 1–49 should have an equal chance of being selected; great pains are taken by the organizers to make sure this is so and far be it from us to suggest it is not totally random. However, Moore (1991) gives an excellent example of a physical, supposedly random, drawing of balls from a bowl in considering the US draft lottery for Vietnam in 1970. This was to be done by birthdate so all the dates in January were put in capsules and were mixed, followed by mixture of these with dates in February and so on with December last. It transpired that, when all the dates were in, the December dates were still mostly on top and far too many dates in December were drawn early than should have happened by chance. This was rather unfortunate for men born in December who were, therefore, much more likely to have lower draft numbers and so be sent to Vietnam earlier ....

However, using a simple random sample means that you are unlikely to incur bias in your results. Our preassessment satisfaction survey was a form of simple random sample. Our sample frame was constructed by listing everybody who passed through the preoperative assessment clinic during a certain time period and a sample was randomly selected. Caution must be exercised when picking people in this manner and checks made that there is no seasonal variation, i.e. there is no reason why people might attend at one period of the year rather than another. Sampling people in the street of a seaside town would give you a different type of population in the winter from in the summer. It also relies on a high percentage of willing respondents. Remember, our sample should be representative of the population as a whole (i.e. everybody who passes through the preoperative assessment clinic).

3.6.5 Systematic random sampling

If at this point we reminded you that for the first stage of our LLI project we sampled 4000 people from the general practice concerned, you might suddenly think of the consequences of using a random number table to select the sampled units. After all, reading the next number carefully, selecting the appropriate unit and repeating the process until 4000 units have been selected is likely to be (1) time-consuming, (2) tedious, (3) increasing the chances of error and (4) likely to leave you with numbers floating across your eyes and nightmares involving random numbers tables.

Systematic sampling can make things much easier; however you do need a complete sample frame. Once more, the sample units need to be numbered on the sample frame from 1 to N (which is the study population size). If we let (as convention dictates) n equal the sample size, then simply divide N by n, i.e. the population size by the required sample size, and call that number k. If k is not a whole number, then round **down** to the nearest whole number. Then randomly select one unit from the first k units on the sample frame (by using a random numbers table or a computer program or whatever) and then select every kth unit.

An example will make this procedure clearer:

Let the population size, N, be 150.
Let the required sample size, n, be 15.
Therefore, $k = 150 / 15 = 10$.

Randomly select one unit from the first 10; let us say this was 3.
Then select every 10th unit.

This gives us, for our sample, units numbered 3, 13, 23, 33, 43, 53, 63, 73, 83, 93, 103, 113, 123, 133 and 143. Counting these confirms we have our 15 sample size.

If our sample size had required to be 14, then k would have equalled 10.71 (150 / 14). Rounding to the nearest number would have given us a value for k equal to 11. If our first randomly selected unit turned out to be higher than unit 7 we would then only have 13 sampled units instead of the required 14 (go on, check it). By always rounding down, we will always get at least the required sample size. Actually, whatever the number of the first unit selected when rounding down, we would end up with a sample size of 15 rather than 14 in this case, but is better to select one too many rather than one too few.

The elderly sample in a particular area of London was selected in this manner. The required sample size was 750 from a population of 53 500. This gave a k of 71 and resulted in 753 people being selected. The LLI study was slightly different in that 4000 people were required from the study population of 6066. As this is around two-thirds of the study population, k was set to 3 and 2022 people were selected, who were then rejected, leaving a final sample size of 4044. Here, therefore, we selected the people who would not be in the sample and surveyed everybody else. k was calculated as 6066 / (6066 − 4000) and rounded up in this case to make sure we were left with at least 4000 people after rejecting those initially selected.

Systematic sampling's main advantages are that it is normally easier than simple random sampling and will save on time and costs.

However, it does have disadvantages. It is not, theoretically, a simple random sample. Not all possible samples of size n have an equal chance of occurring, simply because of the method of selecting the sample. The more major problem is if the list is arranged in any way. Consider a list simply arranged male–female–male–female–male–

female, etc. If k turned out to be 2 or any even number, we would end up selecting only members of one sex. Therefore, before performing systematic sampling, always check for any underlying order in the sampling frame. Actually it may not always be a bad thing to have order in the frame. A sampling frame arranged youngest to oldest, for example, or by address blocks, should give a good spread of ages or locality respectively.

3.6.6 Stratified sampling

Think back, if you will, to our survey of elderly people in a district of London. Imagine that the district could be neatly split into three, not necessarily equal, localities (say, for simplicity's sake, electoral wards). Now these wards, we discovered by analysing national Census data, have completely different Townsend deprivation index scores and tend to be inhabited by people from different social classes (which we can measure by considering their occupation). Ward 1 could be considered a very affluent area and mainly social classes 1 and 2 (the highest social classes); ward 2 around the norm for the UK as a whole, mainly social class 3; and ward 3 a more deprived area with social class 4 and 5. Now, you suspect that their different levels of deprivation would lead to different results for your main question of your survey. For example, rates of asthma-like symptoms have been shown to be associated with deprivation (Eachus *et al.*, 1996). Taking the population as a whole would cover up information of the individual electoral wards. So, what we can do is divide the whole study population into subpopulations (here based on electoral wards) so each person in the study population is in one subpopulation. We can then simply take a random sample from each subpopulation. Our electoral wards (or subpopulations) are called **strata** and this is stratified random sampling.

However, this is only suitable when, in terms of the characteristic under investigation, the strata differ widely from each other but within each stratum the variation is very low. The next subsection will look at a form of sampling when the subpopulations are assumed (maybe from evidence in secondary data) to be very similar in terms of the characteristic under investigation.

The advantage of stratified sampling is that it gives more precise knowledge of the subpopulations and will then, provided that the strata are different as stated above, give a better overall estimator for the population as a whole. It may also be administratively convenient to recognize the subpopulations rather than take the population as a whole. However, it does lead to different types of sampling problem, which we will not discuss here but which can be found in the suggested further readings.

Using an ordered list (such as by age or address) in systematic sampling as described earlier is a form of stratification as you are, in effect, stratifying by the characteristic by which the list is ordered. Unordered lists in systematic sampling take on the effect of cluster sampling, which is the next form of sampling we move on to. In systematic sampling we are, in effect, breaking the population down into subpopulations based on the size of k.

3.6.7 Cluster sampling

Cluster sampling needs to be compared to stratified sampling and their differences understood. Stratified sampling is concerned with differences between subpopulations; in cluster sampling we believe that these subpopulations are similar in terms of the characteristic under investigation. These subpopulations are called clusters and should be relatively homogeneous. The selected cluster or clusters can be used to represent the population as a whole.

In cluster sampling, the clusters become like our sampling units. Instead of selecting the unit, or individuals, we select one or more of the clusters to act as the 'representatives' of the population as a whole. So, for example, in our LLI survey, we might have decided that the characteristics of the patients in all the general practices in Stoke-on-Trent were very similar (i.e. for this study, the rates of LLI would be very similar across all practices); we could then have selected, by use of a random numbers table perhaps, one general practice and obtained the results for that practice, assuming that they would be similar to all practices in Stoke. This was not actually the case, as we believed rates of LLI were associated with different levels of deprivation. We are, therefore, not extrapolating our results across the whole of Stoke.

Advantages of cluster sampling are that it is often easier and cheaper than completely simple random sampling. It can also be useful if the sample frame is incomplete (for example, in the more deprived countries you may only have registers for some of the villages in a province). Provided you have no reason to suspect that units not on the frame will be any different from those on it, you can use cluster sampling to represent the whole population.

After selecting your cluster or clusters, you can either survey everyone in the selected clusters or select a sample from them. The latter form is called **multistage sampling.** Stage 1 is selecting clusters, stage 2 is sampling from within these clusters. The sample in stage 2 may be drawn as per a simple random sample or systematic sample, for example. If more than one cluster is selected, then, if they are all of similar size, you may decide to select the same number from each cluster. Alternatively, you may weight the clusters so that people in the bigger clusters have more chance of being selected. This is called sampling with **probability proportional to size (pps).** For more information about pps, see, for example, Barnett, 1991.

The important thing to remember about cluster sampling is that the clusters should be homogeneous, i.e. be similar under the variable that is being investigated.

3.7 SAMPLE SIZE

Possibly the most often asked question concerning a survey is concerned with the sample size. This is the most likely point at which you need to consult a statistician but you should go prepared as s/he will not be able to give you an answer without some information from you first.

The purpose of this section is to give you an idea of what you should be thinking about when deciding on sample size. Too many will waste resources, too few will reduce the accuracy of your data. There is a fallacy that the proportion of sample size to population size (known as the **sampling fraction**) is always important. It is, in fact, only important if the intended sample size is greater than about one-20th of the population size. Calculating sample size is often a compromise between statistical calculation and resources in terms of time, money and manpower. You will need to go back to your main variable (i.e. the variable relating to your main aim) and consider the following points. It is also quite complex and great detail is beyond the scope of this book.

The sample size will be larger:

- the more variable the population is under the chosen characteristic. Obviously, if all the population is very similar then you will not need to survey too many of them to get the information you require. If, however, they are vastly different, you will need to survey a lot more to get a good representation of the population. You can get indications of the variability of your study population from literature reviews, previous similar studies and pilot studies.

- the more accurate you wish to be; how closely would you hope the sample data matches the population data? The more accurate you wish to be, the larger your sample size will need to be. If you are testing drugs you may wish to be extremely accurate, within ± 1% for proportion-measured variables, for example, because of the importance for human suffering. For other studies, you may be happy to be within ± 5%. This is often called the **margin of error**. When considering, for example, the income of doctors at a particular level, you might be happy to be within £2000 of the real mean (average) income, or, maybe, you would prefer to be within £100.

- the more confident you wish to be that there is this accuracy. We have already told you that you can never be certain in statistics (as in life) and again, depending on the survey, we may be happy to be 95% confident about the accuracy of our data. At other times, we may require 99% confidence. We can define 95% confidence as meaning that, if we repeated our survey 100 times on different samples from our population, we would be within the required accuracy on 95 of those occasions.

- if you are considering differences on a characteristic between subdivisions of a population then the smaller the difference you expect to find, and the more confidence you want that there is this difference, the bigger the sample size must be.

There are tables (e.g. Table 3.6; we shall return to this shortly) and computer programs available to calculate sample size. See Florey, 1993 for the ideas behind the more basic sample size calculation formulae. Lwanga and Lemeshow (1991) have produced tables of sample size calculations but it would be worthwhile reading Chapters 5–8 in this text before referring to their text. Do not be put off by the fact that we surveyed 4000 people in our LLI survey. We needed to do this as we were filtering people off during the first stage. For some surveys you may only need a handful of people. As stated previously, it can be a compromise between statistical precision and resources to hand. Increasing the sample size to the detriment of the quality of the rest of the study design may not be worthwhile. It may well be a case of reducing the precision you can get from your study in order to make sure that the smaller study is done well. For stratified and multistage sampling you will need to consider how many people you will need to select from each subgroup and for all surveys, how you are going to analyse the data.

Table 3.6 gives us sample sizes for estimating population proportions with an estimated proportion of 0.5 (that is one-half of the population) having the characteristic under study.

Table 3.6

Example of sample size calculations for population proportions: minimum sample sizes needed when estimated population proportion is 0.5 with different levels of accuracy and confidence, e.g. to be within 5% of the population proportion with 95% confidence, you would need a sample size of at least 385 (Based on table in Biles, 1995)

| | Minimum sample size | | |
Margin of error	90% confidence	95% confidence	99% confidence
±5%	271	385	664
±4%	423	601	1037
±3%	752	1068	1842
±2%	1692	2401	4148
±1%	6766	9604	16577

A figure of 0.5 will give us the largest necessary sample size and can be used as our estimate when we have little or no knowledge of the real population proportion. For a confidence level of 95% and a margin of error of ± 5% we see we need a sample size of 385 (which we could round up to 400). If we had used the proportion of people with LLI from the 1991 Census in Stoke-on-Trent (around 24% or 0.24) then we would only have needed to sample around 280 people (from Table 1 in Lwanga and Lemeshow, 1991). Other tables and computer programs will give sample sizes for comparing between groups or estimating means (averages).

3.8 SOURCES OF ERROR

We have already occasionally mentioned errors that can creep into surveys. We shall now look a little closer at the sources of these errors so that you know what your enemy is in the survey battlefield.

There are two main types of error: **sampling error** and **non-sampling error**. Sampling error is the difference between results obtained from taking a sample and results obtained from taking a complete census. Random sampling errors are the natural effect of taking a sample rather than a census and it is difficult to reduce this. The beauty of statistics is that it helps you quantify and display the potential size of this random error, as we shall discover later in the text. We shall look at the meaning of sampling error again in Chapter 7.

Non-sampling error is the difference between results from a complete census and the correct results, i.e. errors that would occur whether you performed a sample survey or a census. It is the non-random sampling error and non-sampling error that we should be most concerned with and these can be broken down into two types; **non-observational error** and **observational error**. These errors can make our results just plain wrong, or even bias them in favour of a particular subset of the population.

3.8.1 Non-observational error

These fall under two headings; **non-inclusion** and **non-response**. Non-inclusion occurs when you give some members of your population no chance of being selected. For example, imagine a survey of people with asthma-like symptoms resident in a district. You decided to take as your study population everyone who attended one of the general practices in the district with asthma-like symptoms within the previous 6 months. By doing this, you would give people with asthma-like symptoms who had not been to their GP in that time period, or presented with unrelated symptoms, or who attended a practice outside the district even though they lived within the district, absolutely no chance of being selected, hence giving a mis-representation of your target population. Therefore, care must be taken when selecting your study population and when relating results to a wider population than your study population actually is.

Non-response can be a particular problem and occurs when people (or units) selected for a sample do not yield data; either refusing to be interviewed, not returning questionnaires or, at a lower level, leaving out some questions.

There are a number of options available to try and reduce non-response; some of the most common are mentioned below.

- For postal surveys, reminders (in the form either of a postcard reminding the recipient about the survey or another copy of the questionnaire) to non-respondents should be sent. Usually at least one is needed. Typically the first reminder after about 3–4 weeks is a postcard and the second, 3–4 weeks after that, another copy of the questionnaire.

- If reminders fail, then telephoning respondents or calling on them personally is a possibility.

- In face-to-face interviews that involved randomly visiting houses, then calling back on another day and at a different time of day is worth a try.

- If the above three options are made impossible by a lack of time and resources, then it may still be worth subsampling the non-respondents and 'blitzing' just those selected for this subsample.

Non-response may happen for a number of reasons and can often be reduced before the study with careful crafting of the questionnaire and covering letter. Apathy on behalf of the respondent means there must be a good covering letter explaining the potential benefits of the research; fears of confidentiality should be allayed also in the letter; personal questions should be piloted beforehand; badly crafted questionnaires will be a turn-off for respondents as will impolite letters or questionnaires. Be careful to make sure that the questions are relevant and clear (see next chapter for questionnaire construction guidance). Always include a stamped addressed envelope for return. Some studies even include gift vouchers for popular stores for those who reply promptly.

Non-response will always occur so an important issue is to try to give the reader or user of your survey an estimate of whether the non-response is important or not.

The response rate (percentage of selected sample that responded) is often used as a sign of the success of a survey. A lot of people will only take account of surveys with at least a 65% response rate but response rates as low as 40–50% can be accurate provided the non-respondents are no different in their characteristics from respondents. So, if possible, get as much information on non-respondents as possible. Do they tend to differ to respondents in terms of age? sex? social class? area of residence? ethnicity? type of occupation? illness? ... Are the results of your survey similar to expectations? Similar to previous surveys? (although, of course, even if they are dissimilar this does not mean they are wrong). In short, is there any reason to think your results would be greatly different if the non-respondents had replied?

3.8.2 Observational errors

There are three common types of observational error; **response error, measurement error** and **recording error**. Response errors occur either through the respondent giving a false answer or due to misunderstanding of the question. This, again, implies the need for a good questionnaire. Measurement error can happen: for example, by measuring blood pressure or a pulse incorrectly or by rounding of numbers to the nearest whole number. Recording errors are, as it sounds, answers that are recorded wrongly, coded wrongly or entered on to a spreadsheet, or similar, wrongly. Care must be taken at all times.

3.9 SUMMARY

This chapter has considered the various steps needed to design an effective and successful survey. Just as poor analysis of quality data can ruin a survey, so can poor data well analysed. This chapter can also be used to allow you to run a critical eye over articles in journals and newspapers reporting studies. Have they stated their methodology? Are they trying to hide anything? Have they explained the reasons behind their methodology? Do not accept that, just because a study has been published, it is a good study.

4 QUESTIONNAIRE DESIGN

4.1 INTRODUCTION

Everybody gets asked at some time in their life whether they 'like their work' but what is not often realized is how vague and ambiguous this question really is. It would be a very lucky person who liked (or do we mean enjoy?) everything about his/her work, so it would be difficult to answer this question in anything but general terms. Further, answering 'no' to this question may not mean that we dislike our work: we may simply put up with it as being something that has to be done. What do we mean by 'work' anyway? The assumption may be the work we do for a living, our paid work. But students and housewives and volunteers work without being paid and do we separate our 'salaried' work from working in the garden, or around the house, or decorating (which may be hobbies for some people)? Furthermore, does the question refer to the actual process of doing the work or the end result of that process? Nurses may not enjoy every aspect of their daily routine but they are likely to get some satisfaction on seeing a once more healthy person leave their ward.

This simple example emphasizes the importance of being absolutely clear and unambiguous with the questions involved in a survey. There is nothing more frustrating and embarrassing than wasting time and money on a large survey only to find that the questions have not been formulated properly or tested rigidly and the answers are meaningless because of mistakes in the question. The importance of piloting (i.e. testing) the questionnaire is often ignored and can lead to disastrous consequences, with options being left out of multiple choice questions, questions implying a certain answer and questions with more than one meaning; all of which could have been discovered and properly corrected if the time to test the questionnaire had been taken before commencing the study. Make sure you can actually get the answers to the questions; that the respondents are **willing** and **able** to give you the answers. One problem with patient-satisfaction-type surveys, for example, is that patients may be unwilling to be critical of doctors or nurses whom they might perceive as being overworked and rushed.

There are many books that give guidance on questionnaire design. Most research design books or sample survey books include chapters on questionnaire design, while books devoted exclusively to the art of questionnaire design include Streiner and Norman, 1995 (concentrating on health), Sudman and Bradburn, 1983 and Foddy, 1993. Also worth consulting are Chapters 5 and 6 from Fowler, 1993. Dixon and Long (1995) and McDowell and Jenkinson (1996) discuss how to select or develop health-related questionnaires.

Words often used instead of questionnaire are 'instrument' and 'tool'. For our purposes, these words can be considered to be synonymous. In this chapter we will discuss some of the key issues concerning questionnaire design but refer to the above texts for more detailed treatment.

4.2 RELIABILITY, VALIDITY AND RESPONSIVENESS

4.2.1 Reliability

Imagine your feelings if you weighed yourself on a set of weighing scales, stood quietly by the side of them for 5 minutes and then weighed yourself again and found that the second time it showed you weighed 2 kg more than the first time. You would be likely to question the accuracy of the scales. Similarly with a questionnaire: if you asked someone to fill in a questionnaire and then fill it in again a day later, you would expect very similar answers the second time around provided nothing had happened in the intervening 24 hours that affected any of the answers. This asset, the ability to produce the same result over time without change in external factors, is called **reliability** and you would expect a questionnaire to possess it.

The most obvious way to check for reliability is to repeat the test and compare results; the test–retest method. This is, of course, time-consuming and an alternative approach is to measure the internal consistency of the questionnaire. This means that similar items (questions) should yield similar results: for example, the Short Form-36 (SF-36) questionnaire can be split into eight different scales of health including general health, physical functioning and mental health. Questions on each scale should be correlated: for example, in general, if someone reported difficulty walking then you might also expect them to have difficulty climbing stairs. This is called **internal consistency** and can be measured using Cronbach's α (see Streiner and Norman, 1995 for more details). Most standard questionnaires used a number of times by different people will be rigorously checked for reliability. For your purposes, comparing answers on similar topics and performing a small test–retest analysis during piloting (covered in section 4.9) should suffice.

4.2.2 Validity

Validity simply means that the question measures what it is supposed to measure, i.e. that the questionnaire (or tool) measures what it is intended to do. There are many different versions of validity and here we shall concentrate briefly on the three main types.

Content validity implies that the wording of items, and the items themselves, represent what the instrument is supposed to measure adequately. The easiest way to measure this is by scrutiny by experts or through careful piloting. For example, for studying the effects of the prevalence of a particular disease on normal daily activities, it would be beneficial to obtain the views of both the medical experts on the illness and the sufferers themselves.

Criterion validity is tested by comparing the instrument against a gold standard under the assumption that they should provide similar results. The new instrument should prove itself to be a more than adequate replacement for the gold standard: perhaps it is easier to use or more acceptable to the study population or more efficient and time-saving. This, of course, assumes that there is a gold standard in the first place! The scales on the SF-36 have been tested against other general health profile questionnaires, such as the Nottingham Health Profile, and more specific illness questionnaires, such as the Shortened Arthritis Impact Measurement Scales (Ware *et al.*, 1993).

Construct validity tests the instrument against previous hypotheses and by deciding what is plausible and what is not. This is, perhaps, a more controversial measure of validity. For example, you might expect those from a higher socioeconomic class to score better on the SF-36. However, this measure of validity relies on your prior beliefs being correct and having a valid measure of socioeconomic class.

4.2.3 Responsiveness

Responsiveness in an instrument means that it has the ability to detect change. A successful health intervention should be apparent from the results of a post-intervention questionnaire compared to the same questionnaire applied before the intervention. Responsiveness is a crucial quality if an instrument is to be used as an outcome measure and is one of the main reasons why the SF-36 is still being debated as an outcome tool even though its effectiveness as a simple general health profile tool has, by and large, been accepted. A slightly different measure of responsiveness (or **sensitivity**) is the ability to distinguish between two groups; perhaps a population with a particular illness and the general population.

4.3 SEARCHING FOR EXISTING QUESTIONNAIRES

There is no point in reinventing the wheel, or even the health questionnaire. One way to get around designing your own questionnaire and the problems that will arise is to use another questionnaire, which should have already been validated and reliability ensured. There are countless health questionnaires around at the moment, ranging from general health profiles to tools for specific diseases. Many, including those mentioned here, are reviewed in texts by Bowling (1994, 1997) and by Wilkin *et al.* (1992). Fitzpatrick (1991a, b) looks at designing surveys and questionnaires for patient satisfaction surveys. However, any questionnaire will always be open to criticism and health-related questionnaires are particularly difficult to construct. The difficulties associated with health questionnaires and suggestions for guidelines in constructing them are discussed by McDowell and Jenkinson (1996). Another method of searching for existing questionnaires is to trawl the literature to discover similar studies to your proposed one. It should then be possible to contact the research team involved and obtain information on any problems they had and copies of the questionnaire used. Databases that can be searched will depend, obviously, on your particular project but popular health- and medicine-related ones are Medline (an American database), HELMIS (based at the Nuffield Institute for Health at the University of Leeds) and BIDS (Bath). A further advantage of using an existing questionnaire, apart from the time and costs it will save, is that it will give you data to compare your results against.

Even if there is no definitive standard questionnaire you can use, it may still be possible to 'lift' questions from other questionnaires. The Centre for Applied Social Surveys (CASS), based at the University of Surrey, is attempting to standardize commonly asked questions, and has a Question Bank that comprises questions from surveys such as the national Census, the British Household Panel Survey and the British Labour Force Survey; this will allow surveyors to directly compare with other surveys. Demographic-type questions can be extracted from the decennial Census; health profile tools like the Short Form-36 and the Sickness Impact Profile (or the British equivalent, the Functional Limitations Profile) can provide questions relating to effect of health on functioning; and more specific questions can be lifted from disease-specific questionnaires.

However, there are difficulties in using an existing questionnaire. Make sure that it was found to be valid and reliable (and responsive if it is to be used as an outcome measure). Also, determine and correct any problems encountered (few studies take place without some problem or other). Make sure that it is suitable for your needs; it may have been prepared for a different purpose and so some questions may not be suitable and changes may still need to be made. Piloting is still a good idea, particularly if the questionnaire has only been used once or twice before, if changes have been made to it or if it was designed for a different population.

4.4 THE DESIGN PROCESS

4.4.1 Art and design

The process of constructing a questionnaire can be considered as more of an art than a science. It would not be going too far to suggest that the questionnaire designer needs to get into the minds of his/her study population. Knowledge of potential respondents and the subject matter is extremely important as you need to know what level to aim the questionnaire at and the respondents' willingness and ability to answer your questions. You do not want to use unfamiliar words; most people do not want to appear unintelligent and so will not admit to ignorance of technical or unusual terms or words. An oft-quoted example of people unwilling to admit ignorance is recorded in Churchill (1987), where a public opinion survey resulted in 99.7% giving an opinion, either positive or negative, on a Metallic Metals Act. This might appear to show a healthy interest in the subject by the public if it was not for the fact that this Act was completely fictional! Some people even include a fictional question like this in their questionnaire as a type of validation for the tool as a whole. The last thing you want is for people to start guessing what a question means. You want people's views to emerge without imposing barriers.

People with past experience of designing questionnaires will be able to give you guidance on what seems to work and what does not and piloting is crucial, but perhaps the most essential element needed will be common sense. In truth, the majority of the art of the questionnaire design is really just common sense, thinking about the subject matter and the people who will be answering your questions. Do not distance yourself from the study population. Include in the design process (as well) experts in the field of the study subject so that the meaning of the question can be made clear.

4.4.2 Deciding on data required

When starting a questionnaire design you need to go back to your research proposal and remind yourself of the main questions you are seeking to answer. Ensure that every question can be used. It is very easy and all too tempting to include questions because they 'seem interesting' or 'might throw up something good' even if they have little to do with the main aims of the study. Before long, your questionnaire will begin to approach the length of *War and Peace*. Remember, the longer the questionnaire and/or the longer it takes to answer it, the less the respondent is likely to want to answer it. Including too many questions will not only reduce the response, it will push up the costs. However, asking too few questions is negligent. There is a fine line between too many and too few questions ...

What also needs to be done at this stage is consideration of the analysis of the questionnaire. Do not leave it until you have a mountain of completed questionnaires in front of you. If you wish to compare respondents by age, sex, ethnicity, locality or some other factor, then, if you have not got the information to hand already, you will need to ask for it on the questionnaire. You also need to consider data entry methods, something which will be discussed further in Chapter 5.

Finally, start selecting the specific items you wish to include that will need to be turned into questions, ensuring each can be used and that the respondents have the ability, willingness and memory (if relevant) to answer each.

4.5 TYPES OF QUESTION

4.5.1 Opinion or factual?

There are two types of question, which seek out different forms of information. The first is the **factual** question, which simply asks for a fact, e.g. age, sex or income. However, although this seems the simplest form of question, care must still be taken to convey precisely what you want to know. For example, if we asked a university student aged 24 years and 8 months (ignoring the days, hours, minutes) his age, he might (quite legitimately) answer any of the following:

24, 24 and a half, coming up to 25, 24 and 8 months, 25 next January, mid-20s.

So, asking what the age was last birthday might be a way round it, or asking for age in the format of years and months. Where the specific age is unimportant, asking the respondent to tick the relevant age group (e.g. 20–34) could be a solution.

Another form of question is the opinion question, which asks respondents their opinion about a topic. These can be of the form 'What do you think about ...' or 'What is your view on ...' or 'Do you believe ...' or 'How did you feel ...'. In these questions, there is no one correct answer so there is a problem in validating the question. Problems with these forms of question are the level of intensity and the relevance of the question. Does the respondent actually care? Two respondents may give the same answer to a question but while one may feel passionately on the subject the other may have selected one option without any great commitment. Someone may care passionately about the introduction of charges for using the hospital car park if they regularly travel there by car, but someone else who always uses public transport may not care so greatly. The final problem is that opinion questions are very sensitive to the actual wording and any emphasis in it, either in the question itself or included by the interviewer in a face-to-face situation. This may lead to bias being incorporated into the question; more of which will be discussed later.

In terms of the limiting long-term illness (LLI) study, the question on having an LLI or not is a subjective, opinion question, and the SF-36 questions are opinion questions, namely opinions about people's own health. Questions on the demographic questionnaire put alongside the SF-36 tend to be factual questions concerning marital status, home ownership, employment status and use of various health services, for example.

4.5.2 Open or closed?

Aside from the straightforward factual question (such as the age question given above), there are two main structures of question. **Closed questions** are multiple-choice-type questions where the respondent has to tick the category most appropriate for him/her. **Open questions** leave a space or a few lines where the respondent can enter whatever s/he wants. A simple example of the two structures is given in Table 4.1.

Again there is no easy choice as to which type of structure to use. It depends on a number of factors, including the actual aim of the question, the format (whether face-to-face or postal) and the type of analysis required. The various advantages and disadvantages of these two structures will now be discussed and are highlighted in Table 4.2. Not all these advantages and disadvantages are invariably valid, however!

With open-ended questions there is no presumption about the response and respondents are left to express their answer in their own words, which is likely to be enjoyed by some respondents more than others; the less literate may struggle with open-ended questions and

Table 4.1 Example of an open and a closed question	**Open** How do you feel about paying to use the hospital car park? .... **Closed** Do you agree with the decision to introduce paying for using the hospital car park? 1) Yes ☐ 2) No ☐ 3) Don't know ☐

	Open	Closed
Table 4.2 Open or closed?	No presumption about response Express in own words Get more information Level of information is known Can develop closed responses Salient points Strength of feelings	Anticipate answers, classify accordingly Multiple choice or rank Easier data entry Easier to compare/analyse Less variable answers Easier to answer (recognition task) Better response?

the less enthusiastic may be disinclined to answer or to answer fully – again, it is important to know your audience.

Supporters of open-ended questions suggest that you get more information as you obtain all the salient points in the respondent's mind, and you get to know how much they actually know and the strength of their feelings; all of which you cannot get from a closed question. However, this does depend on all respondents being enthusiastic and interested enough to answer fully. The stress of a face-to-face interview may also mean that the respondent 'forgets' information or does not answer as fully as s/he would have done given more time. There is, in any case, a limit to the number of open-ended questions one can ask. While there must be a limit to the number of closed questions it is possible to ask as well, open-ended questions will be harder work for the respondent and more time-consuming in the administration, whether postal or face-to-face.

For closed questions the answers have to be anticipated beforehand and classified accordingly. A possible way around this is to use open-ended questions for the pilot survey and then closed questions based on the answers for the main survey. In any case, the pilot survey should reveal any missing categories. A fail-safe is to include an 'other' option which the respondent ticks if none of the other choices apply to him/her and a gap for the 'other' to be explained. It may be possible to develop closed responses from open-ended questions after the survey but it is time-consuming and will lose much of the richness of the data collected by this method.

Closed questions can be simple multiple-choice or can be options to be ranked in order of preference or salience (giving the options weightings). Closed questions can be easier to enter into a spreadsheet or other computer package and the less variable answers make them easier to analyse. They are easier to answer as well: it is simply a 'recognition' task for the respondent as to which option is most suitable for him/her and, in this way, it is likely to give a better response. A possible 'middle line' is to use closed categories with an optional space for any comments the respondents might have, although, again, time and space will reduce the number of questions it is possible to do this on.

Closed questions will allow the quantitative analysis discussed in this book while open-ended questions are more in the line of qualitative work (unless the answers are categorized at a later stage). Open-ended questions are best for semi-structured and unstructured interviews and need a competent and highly trained interviewer to prompt and follow up if necessary in a face-to-face setting.

The SF-36 and demographic questionnaire in the LLI project comprise all closed questions with an option to comment at the end of the SF-36 and 'other' categories being included with some additional space for comments at the end of certain questions on the demographic questionnaire. Likewise, the hospital satisfaction survey questionnaire contains closed questions with 'other' options and comments encouraged after some questions.

4.5.3 Response scales for closed questions

As you can probably gather from the previous section, the options available in closed questions are all-important to make the question a successful one. For factual questions, it is simply a case of listing all possible answers with a final option for an 'other' with a 'please state' alongside it to cater for ones you had not thought of; if you do not include an 'other' category, then you have to ensure that the options are exhaustive. This is similarly the case for motivation-type questions. For example, alternative answers to the question 'Why did you not ask the nurses on the ward about any concerns you had?' could include 'Had no concerns', 'The nurses seemed too busy', 'Did not seem important', 'Did not feel questions were encouraged', 'Preferred to ask the doctor' and 'Other – please state'.

It is also important to make clear whether the respondent is supposed to tick one box, is allowed to tick all that apply or is supposed to rank in order of importance. For example, consider the question and its possible answers below:

4 Questionnaire design

'Which of the following do you believe are important features of a good out-patient service? Please tick the boxes of all that apply.'

a)   public transport available to and from service ☐

b)   short waiting times ☐

c)   cheap refreshments ☐

d)   high quality refreshments ☐

e)   plentiful seating ☐

f)   efficient appointments system ☐

The respondent is allowed to tick as many or as few as s/he wishes. However, s/he is likely to believe that one feature is more important than another that s/he selects (perhaps believing that short waiting times are most important, followed by plentiful seating and then good public transport). There will be no indication of this weighting from the answer to this question. However, asking the respondent to rank all that apply with '1' indicating the most important will add more information. Including a 'Please comment' section will allow the respondent to elucidate on his/her answer as well. In contrast, asking what types of vaccination a person has had obviously would be non-sensical to rank.

A special type of opinion question is the attitude question, which asks people to consider various statements and their reaction to them. For example, we might ask how much the respondent agreed with the statement that the hospital food was appetizing and use the scale:

a) strongly agree

b) agree

c) neutral

d) disagree

e) strongly disagree

This type of balanced scale is called a **Likert scale**. An unbalanced scale considering the question about the taste of hospital food might have options:

a) absolutely disgusting

b) disgusting

c) awful

d) not very good

e) fair

This, rather extreme, example immediately creates the impression in the respondent's mind that the food cannot be very nice as the scale is so weighted in that way. However, the options should be balanced equally between positive and negative. An alternative to the first Likert example is:

a) very satisfied

b) satisfied

c) dissatisfied

d) very dissatisfied

which could be used for an appropriate situation. Notice this last scale has no 'middle' option; we could have included a 'neutral' (or 'neither satisfied nor dissatisfied') or a 'don't know' or 'undecided' to this scale (or even more than one, as they have different meanings). Including a middle option is down to the aim of the question; if we are measuring strong tendencies we would include a middle option so we would only get positive or negative answers that were strongly held; if we were measuring leanings then we would leave out a middle option to force people to respond either positively or negatively. The problem with the latter, as with all closed questions, is that people may miss out the question if the option they most associate with is not there. By and large, the middle option is included.

The order of the options can also be important and they should be varied (i.e. sometimes the positive options go first, sometimes the negative) throughout the questionnaire to allow for discovery of any possible trends, e.g. people just ticking the first or second option each time rather than reading, and thinking about, each question.

An important element of questionnaire design is to keep the respondent interested. One way of doing this is to vary the type of scale used. Some others commonly used include pictures; for example a very happy, smiley face for very satisfied moving down through a happy, neither happy nor sad, sad and, finally, a very sad face for very dissatisfied. Some, such as asking the respondent to indicate a point on a line between the two extremes (e.g. very satisfied and very dissatisfied) where they feel is most appropriate, are very difficult to analyse. If you are going to create your own scale, consider, firstly, how you will analyse it.

4.6 WORDING

Again, a lot of the composing of the actual questions is down to common sense and we shall only briefly highlight the main areas where a question can become unstuck.

4.6.1 Ambiguity

Do not use words that are unspecific. Words like 'frequently', 'normally' and 'occasionally' are likely to mean different things to different people. Try and use specific time periods rather than these terms, as we will discuss shortly. Even the word 'unemployed' is not specific (as various governments' attempts to change its definition prove!). Also, avoid words that have more than one meaning. The word 'theatre' will have different primary meanings for doctors and actors; 'football' will have a different meaning depending on whether you are talking to an Englishman (association football) or an American (American football) – and it can also be used to mean rugby football as well! Different sections of the population may interpret the same word differently. A word that appears to have a straightforward definition may have a slang alternative for some sections of the community.

4.6.2 Understandable

This subsection is normally subtitled 'When in Rome, speak as the Romans do'. If you are surveying the general population then you really need to step into their shoes and decide what they will, and will not, understand. We have already said that most people will not want to admit to ignorance so be careful about those technical words you use as everyday language at work that are rarely used elsewhere. Just as non-cricket-lovers are likely to be bamboozled by cricketing terms like 'silly mid off', 'square leg' and 'the wrong 'un', most people will be confused when presented with many medical terms and phrases. If you have to use a technical word, consider including an explanation of it. On the other hand, if you are directing your questionnaire to professionals in that particular field, then they may feel insulted at 'simple' language being used instead of the correct term, or by explanations alongside the term.

It is essential the question is clear, concise and understandable. Your results will be pointless if people are guessing at the meaning of words or interpreting the question in different ways. In the same vein, it is important that the questions are understandable; try answering the following question quickly: 'Do you agree or disagree that the local hospital should not be closed down?' For this question it is very easy to find yourself giving the opposite answer to the one you intend if you are not careful.

4.6.3 Avoid biased or loaded questions

Consider the following question: 'Do you agree that something should be done about the underspending on the National Health Service (NHS)?' This is a loaded question. It implies that there is underspending on the NHS and, faced with this question, the vast majority will agree that something should be done about it. But, just think how the tabloid newspapers would react to the answers to this question – '95% believe more should be spent on the NHS!!!'; 'NHS seen as priority for funding by general population'. This may well be the truth, but consider the different answers that would be got if the question was instead: 'Do you believe that money should be taken out of education and job creation and put into health?'

4.6.4 Double-barrelled questions

Avoid questions that actually contain more than one question. The following question is actually a double-barrelled question: 'During your stay in hospital, did you feel comfortable asking doctors and nurses questions?' If you were answering this question and you felt comfortable asking doctors questions but not the nurses (or vice versa) then you would be stuck if you could only tick one box. So, in constructing your questionnaire, make sure that all the questions are precise. Also, make sure they are concise: you do not want long rambling questions in which the respondent has forgotten how it started by the time s/he finishes the question.

4.6.5 Time periods

Be careful about specifying periods. Foddy (1993) reports a study from 1965 about the effects of elapsed time on memory of hospitalization, something most people would tend to remember. In the first 10 weeks after discharge, only 3% of hospitalization cases were forgotten by respondents; this rose to 6% for the next 10 weeks and reached a staggering 42% a year after the event. If the time period is too far back, then there may be problems for the respondent remembering. Also, be consistent: do not change the time periods throughout the questionnaire and think carefully about what this time period should be. The SF-36 uses the previous 4 weeks to assess health. For our demographic questionnaire, we decided that the previous 3 months was a long enough time to measure use of common health services such as the GP or chiropodist.

Instead of specifying time periods where people have to work out exactly how far back they need to go (e.g. what was the date 3 months ago?), it may be possible to use landmark events, e.g. 'since Christmas' or 'since the start of term' for surveys of students. This should make it easier for respondents to visualize the time period required.

4.7 EXAMPLES OF CONSTRUCTING QUESTIONS

Take a look at the following four questions and try and redesign them so that they are more precise and informative. Also, think about coding and presentation. Then look at how these questions were asked in different surveys; the first three are taken from the SF-36 health profile tool, the last from the hospital satisfaction survey.

Questionnaire I

Question 1
Have you been in pain recently?

Tick one

YES ☐

NO ☐

Question 2
Has pain interfered with your work?

Tick one

YES ☐

NO ☐

Question 3
Do you have problems with any of the following (tick all that apply)?

a) climbing several flights of stairs ☐

b) climbing one flight of stairs ☐

c) walking half a mile ☐

d) walking one hundred yards ☐

Question 4
If you had a test while in hospital, did you find the explanation of the purpose of the test easy or difficult to understand?

Easy ☐

Difficult ☐

The actual questions (questions 1–3) used for these topics on the SF-36 are:

Question 1 – Revised
How much **bodily** pain have you had during the **past 4 weeks**?

	Circle one
None	1
Very mild	2
Mild	3
Moderate	4
Severe	5
Very severe	6

Question 2 – Revised
During the **past 4 weeks**, how much did **pain** interfere with your normal work (including both work outside the home and housework)?

	Circle one
Not at all	1
A little bit	2
Moderately	3
Quite a bit	4
Extremely	5

Question 3 – Revised
The following questions are about activites you might do during a typical day. Does **your health limit you** in these activities?

	(Circle one number on each line)		
ACTIVITIES	Yes, limited a lot	Yes, limited a little	No, not limited at all
a) Climbing **several** flights of stairs	1	2	3
b) Climbing **one** flight of stairs	1	2	3
c) Walking **half a mile**	1	2	3
d) Walking **one hundred yards**	1	2	3

Obviously, you are likely to have come up with different forms of these questions, which may work just as well as these used on the SF-36. However, for the time being consider these revisions and see if your answers have similar properties.

Firstly, they are more precise than the first attempts. A time period is defined for questions 1 and 2 (rather than the vague term 'recently') and more information is obtained from each question by expanding the possible answers. Question 2 now attempts to define what it means by 'work' while question 3 gives an introduction to the question. Notice also that key words are highlighted by being emboldened.

We hope you also remembered to **code** your answers as the SF-36 has! This makes data entry into a computer so much easier. For example, in question 3, instead of typing 'Yes, limited a little' if the respondent has circled this option, we can just enter '2' into the computer.

Question 4 is really three questions in one and assumes that the patient had a test and that the purpose of it was explained. The actual questions used had filters and excluded blood and urine tests. It could be suggested that they are still quite general questions as they do not specify particular tests or ask the respondent which test(s) they had. They are as follows:

Questionnaire 3

Now a few questions about any tests you may have had.

4. Were you given any **tests** during your stay in hospital other than blood or urine tests?

	Circle one	
Yes	1	Go to question 5a
No	2	Go to question 6
Can't remember/don't know	3	Go to question 6

5a. Was the **purpose** of the tests explained to you by the hospital staff?

	Circle one	
Yes	1	Go to question 5b
No	2	Go to question 6
Can't remember/don't know	3	Go to question 6

5b. Was the explanation easy or difficult to understand?

	Circle one
Very easy	1
Fairly easy	2
Neither easy nor difficult	3
Fairly difficult	4
Very difficult	5
Can't remember/can't say	6

4.8 QUESTIONNAIRE STRUCTURE

The first questionnaire you design is likely to be overlong and slightly unwieldy and will therefore need pruning and to become more attractively presented. Remember, for a postal survey, the questionnaire is all the contact the respondent will have with you and so it needs to be presentable, with instructions clearly explained and easy to follow and not discouraging to the respondent. For face-to-face interviews, you still need the questionnaire to be clear for the interviewer to follow in the more stressful conditions of an interview.

4.8.1 General information

Whether in a postal survey, a letter asking for permission to arrange a time to interview or a request for an immediate interview, a number of important issues have to be raised that the respondent needs to know and understand. They include:

- **confidentiality** – the respondents must not feel restricted in any way in giving their answers. If they feel that the truthful answer might lead to a comeback (maybe in denial of health service access) they are unlikely to answer truthfully or even answer at all. Similarly, they should not feel compelled to answer.

- **reasons for the survey** – surveys are becoming ever more popular, with some sections of the community regularly having questionnaires land on their desk or doormat. For a discussion about poor response rates from general practice surveys see McAvoy and Kaner (1996) and the follow-on commentaries by Lydeard and Springer and van Marwijk. If respondents feel that the only reason for the survey is to allow someone to complete a dissertation, for example, they may be less likely to want to take part. If they feel, however, that the survey results will also lead to a benefit either for them or for some other part of the community they will feel more inclined to answer the questions. Good questionnaire design will also encourage participation. Emphasize the importance of the questions, particularly if they are of a personal nature where people may either resent giving information or come to the wrong conclusion as to why a particular question is asked.

- **reasons why they were selected** – most people are naturally suspicious, and they will wonder why they, in particular, were selected; what characteristics they have got that others have not. You will need to explain, for example, that they were randomly selected from a group of people who all have the following characteristics.

- **who you are and who any collaborators on the study are** – if, for example, you are performing a survey for a local group of GPs, emphasize that you are independent of them, but that they agree with the study.

- **reminder of how to return the form if it is a postal survey** – that is, reminding them to place the completed questionnaire in the prestamped and addressed envelope that you have, of course, supplied with it.

For postal surveys, clear instructions (usually at the top of the questionnaire) on how to complete the form should be given.

4.8.2 Questionnaire layout

Again, much of the design of the layout of questionnaires is down to common sense. Make sure each page of the questionnaire is numbered. For ease of data entry into a computer spreadsheet or statistical package make sure that each option in closed questions is coded as in the example questions in section 4.7 (see also Chapter 5 for more on data entry). Do not crowd the questions on to pages to reduce the total number of pages. If the questionnaire gets too bulky, try to remove some questions rather than jam more on individual pages; this can perhaps be done after the piloting stage, when unsuccessful questions can be discarded. Vary the format of questions to keep a respondent's interest, maybe using different types of closed question as discussed in section 4.5.

Do not start the questionnaire with difficult or personal questions. To start a questionnaire by asking intimate questions about the respondent's sex life or about their thoughts on emotive subjects like euthanasia or the death penalty is unlikely to convince respondents that this is a questionnaire they want to carry on with. They are more likely to be filled with dread as to what else is coming later in the questionnaire. Start with easier, straightforward questions and, if difficult questions have to be asked, build up to them gently. Even if they do not answer these questions, at least they will have answered the majority of the questionnaire first. For more on asking threatening questions, see Sudman and Bradburn (1983).

Try not to use too much re-routing or branching (or filtering as it is sometimes called). By this we mean statements like 'if yes, go to question 5; if no, go to question 15'. When people are sent off all over the questionnaire like a treasure hunt searching for the pot of gold, somewhere in the questionnaire they are apt to answer questions they should not and miss out the ones they should answer. Keep this to a minimum and make the instructions clear. If re-routing is necessary, make sure it is always forward in direction rather than backwards and forwards.

Many people believe that coloured paper makes questionnaires more attractive to the eye. In our experience, white paper is as good as any and at least it is a neutral colour. Respondents may be put off by dazzling yellow or fluorescent orange. Coloured questionnaires may be most appropriate if different types of people have to answer different sections of the questionnaire. So, for example, in a survey of marketing functions within hospital trusts, those with a separate specialized marketing department might be asked to fill in one colour of questionnaire; those without such a department should be asked to fill in a different-coloured questionnaire that has different questions.

To keep the respondent's mind fixed on the particular subjects it is usually best to keep questions on the same topic together, introducing the topic with a heading or a few lines of explanation as to why the questions on that topic are important. Some commentators suggest repeating a question with slightly different wording later on in the questionnaire as a test of the reliability of the question. This, unfortunately, if done too often in the questionnaire, is likely to lead to an unwieldy and unstructured, i.e. messy, questionnaire.

Make sure you leave plenty of room for answers for open-ended questions, or at least enough room to get the length of answer you want. However, think about the length of the questionnaire. A form with the length of a mighty tome will be off-putting to say the least. An overlong questionnaire will lead to a drop in the respondent's morale part way through or respondent fatigue and a consequent fall in the quality of answer.

4.9 PRETESTS AND PILOTING

Piloting your questionnaire is an essential element of a survey. You do not want to commit all your resources to a survey and then find that there are elementary mistakes that could have been ironed out by use of a pilot survey first.

The first thing to do is to pretest on a few colleagues or friends to erase all the obvious mistakes that someone coming fresh to the tool is more likely to notice. These are grammatical or spelling errors and they can also make comments about appearance and ease on the eye. Then, you will need to pilot the questionnaire on a small sample of the study population (NB: the results from the pilot should not be included in your final analysis nor should those surveyed at the pilot stage be included in the final sample). The idea of piloting is to iron out all the design faults such as:

- check for any missing options for closed questions or turn an open question into a closed question by using the answers in the pilot survey;
- check wording for ambiguity, misunderstanding and so on as listed in section 4.6;
- look out for any unusual results from the pilot survey and check to see if this is a fault in the questionnaire or a biased study population or question;
- check the success or not of re-routing; did respondents get confused?
- look at the variability of answers; will the questions inform and can respondents answer the question correctly?

If possible, perform the pilot survey in a face-to-face situation even if the final survey will be performed via the post. Then you can ask the respondents if any of the questions made them feel uncomfortable, whether the instructions were clear, how they interpreted questions (to make sure the questions were interpreted correctly), whether they understood all questions/words, whether some sections dragged or whether they got bored. A good idea would be to ask the respondent to think out loud as they answer each question.

Pilot surveys can give you ideas about final sample size and, most importantly, whether the survey is likely to work as intended or not! You might (although we hope this will not be the case) come to the conclusion that there is no point in going on, that you will not get your answers through use of a survey. At least in this case you have saved yourself the time and costs associated with a full-scale survey.

4.10 SUMMARY

The fact that there are a number of texts devoted solely to question-naire design indicates the importance, and size, of the subject. Only the key areas of what is involved in questionnaire design have been considered but perhaps the most vital elements of questionnaire design are common sense and testing of the questions before the survey gets properly under way. It cannot be overemphasized that questionnaire design is much more complicated than just sitting down and scribbling a few questions on to a piece of paper. Knowledge of the study population, clarity and conciseness are vital. Presentation is also crucial. You should study questionnaires that are given to you to fill in whether they are bank forms, market research questionnaires or whatever, and critically appraise them and think how you would improve them.

5 STARTING THE ANALYSIS

5.1 INTRODUCTION

Although this chapter logically follows on from the previous two, it cannot be emphasized enough that you should start considering data entry and analysis while designing your survey and questionnaire. A bit of thought in the questionnaire, as suggested in the previous two chapters, can make entry of data into the computer easier, while familiarity with software and the required analysis techniques can be sharpened before the time for proper use arrives.

Furthermore, while we have so far been concentrating on sample surveys, the rest of the text becomes a little more general. So, while they are appropriate for sample survey methodology usually involving questionnaires, the analyses discussed can also be used (depending on the assumptions discussed at the relevant stages of the text) for other methods of obtaining data. These include data already collected by other people, data collected over a period of time and data collected from subjects by a third party, e.g. costs of various treatments, nurses collecting data on blood pressure and temperature from patients and clinical trials, which are described more fully in Chapter 11. Indeed, while it is extremely important to have confidence in the accuracy and validity of your data, for any data set the starting point must be the descriptive analyses described in this chapter and the next.

This chapter will briefly consider the various computer statistical packages available as well as data entry and the initial analysis of the data. It also includes the assessment of the quality of the data.

Consideration of the computer software available is crucial: you will need to decide whether you have to purchase any software and whether you require either to teach yourself the use of the software or go on a training course. All this is necessary at an early stage of the investigation. If you are using a postal survey the time when the questionnaires go out and you are waiting for them to return is the ideal opportunity to make yourself familiar with all necessary software. If you are using a different package for data entry from that for analysis you will need to consider whether the two packages are compatible; for example, some statistical packages will import a spreadsheet such as a Microsoft Excel file but others will not. You may have to save files as a third type, such as an ASCII file, or reformat them.

5.2 STATISTICAL SOFTWARE PACKAGES

There are many and varied statistical software packages on the market today: some for general use, some for more specific purposes, some for basic analyses only, some for more advanced analyses. A number of them are Windows-driven (i.e. accessed by pull-down menus), others involve programming skills or, at least, knowledge of relevant commands. The menu-driven packages are the easiest to use and tend to be more user-friendly. Packages like SPSS (Statistical Package for the Social Sciences) for Windows and MINITAB for Windows have all the general analytical tools that you are likely to need. More advanced or specialist packages may involve programming such as GLIM and GEN-STAT. Other commonly used packages include SAS and BMDP, while there is a plethora of other statistical packages on the market including the likes of ARCUS, NCSS and SYSTAT. A complete review would be impossible as new packages are constantly being marketed and existing packages updated (at the time of writing, MINITAB had reached version 11 and SPSS for Windows version 8).

Most statistical packages have free demonstration discs, which you can send off for and try before committing yourself to the 'real thing'.

For simple analyses a spreadsheet may suffice. Microsoft Excel is a spreadsheet contained in the Microsoft Office suite. It is useful in that it contains most simple statistical analyses and Excel files can easily be taken over into other statistical packages such as SPSS for Windows and MINITAB. Lotus 1-2-3 is another commonly used spreadsheet. Also worth a mention is EPI INFO, which is freely available and intended for epidemiological studies. It allows you construct your questionnaire and enter data using the questionnaire form on screen and contains many general analyses (Dean *et al.*, 1995).

Computer packages are getting easier to use and allow much easier handling of data. This includes correcting data entry errors, computing new variables from existing ones, running analyses and quickly producing graphs. However, this also makes it easier to get lost in the maze of analyses available, or to forget about what you are trying to discover with your data and end up following one 'interesting' thought after another.

What is crucial to remember is that it is easy to click on an analysis tool on a menu and get a multitude of impressive-looking results. However, you need to make sure that:

- you are asking the right question, using the correct analysis tool and understanding its assumptions and limitations;
- you understand what the requested analysis does;
- you understand all the output.

If you do not pass these three requirements, then you will not know if the computer is giving you valid and interesting results, or a load of garbage because the original question asked was poor or the selected analysis was not appropriate. You will also be in danger of interpreting the results wrongly.

If you are buying a computer statistical package (and you are unlikely to want to perform the analysis by hand) then you will need to consider the requirements needed for the computer to support it (some packages take up a lot of space on the hard drive of your computer and need large amounts of RAM – random-access memory), the level of advancement to which your analysis requirements run and the on-line help systems and accompanying manuals (the user-friendliness of both of these can vary dramatically). Consult with a statistician as to which package s/he recommends that best suits your needs.

Much of the computer output shown in the rest of this text was produced using SPSS for Windows version 6.1 as this is one of the more popular packages. However, output from other packages should not be too dissimilar.

5.3 DATA ENTRY

Strange as it may sound, it often takes longer to input data than to analyse it, particularly for large sample sizes. It can be a tedious job but it is a vitally important one. It is important not to rush it in the enthusiasm to get on to the more interesting part, i.e. the analysis.

Figure 5.1 is an example of a spreadsheet used for collating answers to the limiting long-term illness survey (although the responses are fictional).

Most, if not all, spreadsheets that can be used for statistical analysis work in the same way. Each respondent has his or her own code (to allow anonymity). As you can see from Figure 5.1, not all respondents have replied; respondent code 1, for example, has not replied. Each respondent has his/her own row or **record**, while the columns are the different variables or **fields**. 'LLI' signifies whether the respondent has an LLI or not (0 = No, 1 = Yes). 'Locality' is the electoral ward they live in (labelled from 1–5, each representing a different electoral ward), age has been entered in years only, for sex 0 = female and 1 = male. The rest of the fields are the scores for the various questions on the Short Form-36 (SF-36), relating to the codes on the questionnaire. So 'SF1' relates to question 1, 'SF3A' to question 3A, and so on. If you look closely, you can see that respondent 23 and respondent 29 have got values of 9.0 for fields SF3C and SF3E respectively. This indicates missing data; i.e. they did not answer these questions.

You should be careful how you treat missing data. Some packages (such as SPSS for Windows) allow you to define variables and the values to be treated as missing data. In the above example, '9.0' was defined as a missing value and is ignored in all analyses automatically by the package. In others, such as Excel, you cannot define missing data values and so care has to be taken in analysis that the number assigned for missing data is not included. In this case, it is probably best to leave the cell blank. If you find variables that regularly have no data, i.e. questions not answered by a large number of respondents, then you should question whether it is worth including that variable in the analysis. Hopefully, however, the piloting stage will have discarded all the questions that obtain poor response rates.

Before beginning input, you must check the formats and individual characteristics of the package you are using, to save having to reformat later.

Many texts on data entry will suggest using two inputters as a check on any errors, but this is very time-consuming and wasteful of man-

Figure 5.1
Example of a spreadsheet

Code	LLI	Locality	Age	Sex	SF1	SF2	SF3A	SF3B	SF3C	SF3D	SF3E	SF3F	SF3G
2	1	1	36	0	4	3	3	3	3	3	3	3	3
3	1	1	39	0	3	2	2	3	2	3	3	3	2
4	1	3	40	0	3	3	2	3	3	2	3	3	3
5	1	1	20	0	4	2	1	2	2	2	2	2	2
7	0	1	67	1	1	4	1	1	1	1	2	1	1
8	1	2	18	1	4	3	3	3	3	3	3	3	3
10	0	4	29	1	3	3	2	2	3	3	3	3	3
12	1	5	20	0	4	3	3	2	3	3	3	3	3
13	1	4	72	0	3	2	2	3	2	3	3	3	3
14	0	2	50	1	4	3	2	3	3	3	3	3	2
15	0	3	45	0	1	4	1	1	1	1	2	1	3
16	0	1	65	1	4	3	2	2	3	3	3	3	3
19	1	1	78	0	4	1	1	2	1	2	3	1	2
20	1	2	43	1	2	4	2	2	2	3	3	3	3
22	1	2	43	1	3	3	1	3	9	2	3	3	2
23	0	2	39	0	2	4	1	3	3	2	3	3	3
24	1	3	43	1	3	3	2	2	2	1	2	2	2
25	0	4	21	0	3	4	1	2	3	1	2	2	2
26	0	5	23	1	3	4	1	2	2	1	2	2	2
27	1	4	62	0	1	5	1	2	2	1	2	2	1
28	0	3	80	0	2	4	1	1	1	2	3	1	1
29	1	2	34	1	2	3	2	3	3	3	3	3	3
32	1	2	36	1	3	3	3	3	3	3	9	3	3
33	0	1	43	1	2	2	2	3	3	3	3	3	3
34	0	3	44	0	2	3	2	3	2	2	3	2	3

power. Often, a glance across the entered data can reveal figures outside the range within which that variable falls. Some computer packages will only allow data entry that is within a preselected specified range, which is an easy way of making sure that data entry outside the legitimate range does not occur. Tables and graphs can also reveal errors, as shown in the later sections of this chapter. However, errors that do not fall outside the expected range of values can be more difficult to detect.

The method we employ is as follows: at the end of each session of data entry (say after every 80 questionnaires inputted) we select a handful, perhaps a quarter, of the questionnaires entered in that session (just take some early entered ones, some later and some in the middle – no need to be too scientific about this) and check that they have been entered correctly. If we find no mistakes in these questionnaires then we are satisfied that mistakes are very rare. If we find only one or two mistakes we might check another quarter to make sure these are rare events. If we find a number of mistakes then we have to conclude that we are having a bad day and check all those entered in that session. This system does not guarantee perfect data entry but should, unless we are very unlucky, ensure that there is not a rash of mistakes. Luckily, checking entry of questionnaire data is a lot quicker than the entry itself. Obviously, if you have time and a small number of questionnaires, then you might check all of them.

5.4 SOME DEFINITIONS

Table 5.1 gives some important definitions for phrases that are commonly used in statistics and will be referred to in articles, papers and texts without recourse to their meaning.

We came across 'variables' to some degree when we considered our sample survey. Remember, we set out to ask many different questions of our sample, with the answers being varied across our study population. A variable is a characteristic of a unit (normally a person) we are

Table 5.1

Some important definitions

Variable	A characteristic of a unit (e.g. an individual) to be measured for all units (individuals) in sample that can vary between units (e.g. height, age, suffering from LLI or not)
Constant	A characteristic that is the same for all units (e.g. in our LLI survey the general practice registered with is a constant)
Statistic	A numerical characteristic of a sample (e.g. proportion, an average of some description)
Univariate data	One variable measured on each unit.
Bivariate data	Two variables measured on each unit
Multivariate data	More than one variable measured on each unit
Dependent variable	The response outcome or result (e.g. presence of LLI or not)
Independent variables	Variables used to explain or predict the dependent variable (e.g. for LLI, independent variables could be socioeconomic variables, locality, age, etc.)
Probability	The likelihood that a particular event will occur

interested in that will vary; compare this to a **constant**, which will be the same (i.e. constant) across all units that we are studying. 'Constant' will feature in our discussion on regression analysis in a slightly different manner in Chapter 10.

In this chapter and in the next, we shall be discussing statistics that will be examined during an analysis. These are normally **summary** measures, summarizing data into a number or numbers such as an average of some kind, a count or a proportion or percentage.

Variables summarized individually are known as univariate data. These can give misleading results if there are other variables that greatly affect them.

The difference between **dependent** and **independent** variables is important; particularly when we start considering the multivariate analyses described in Chapters 9 and 10. The independent variables are used to describe, or explain, the dependent variable. That is, we want to assess how much the value of the dependent variable 'depends' on the values of the independent variable or variables (there may be one or more independent variables). For example, having a limiting long-term illness might be related to lower SF-36 scores, as might being elderly. The SF-36 scale score in this case is the dependent variable and having an LLI or not and age are the independent variables.

Statistics, as you will come to see later when we move on to inferential statistics, uses the word **probability** often. The probability of something happening (for example, of it raining tomorrow) can range from 0 (definitely will not happen) up to 1 (definitely will happen). The closer to 1 we get, the more certain we are of something happening. The closer to zero it is, the smaller the chance of something happening. If we toss a coin, and asked you to call heads or tails, you would have a 1 in 2 or 0.5 (1 divided by 2) probability of calling correctly. The 'something happening' in this case is you calling correctly.

If we asked you to pick a card from a pack of playing cards, we would have a 1 in 52 or 0.019 (1 divided by 52) probability of correctly guessing which card you had chosen. Alternatively, we would have a probability of 51 out of 52 or 0.981 (calculated as 1 – 0.019) of incorrectly guessing your card.

The total probability must sum to 1 when all possible events are included. For example, the probability of picking a heart at random from a pack of cards is ¼. Similarly, the probabilities of picking a club, diamond or a spade are each ¼. These four probabilities sum to 1 as you can only pick either a club, diamond, heart or spade.

5.5 TYPES AND MEASUREMENT SCALES OF DATA

The type of data and scale used to measure it are very important in deciding on the method of analysis, as will be seen later in this chapter and in the rest of the text.

Categorical data is where each sampling unit will fall into one (or more) particular groups (or categories). There are two subtypes of measurement for such data: **nominal**, where there is no particular order to the categories, and **ordinal**, where there is an order to the categories. Sex, where, for example, '0' signifies female and '1' signifies male and locality (labelled, perhaps, from '1' upwards, each number representing different localities) are examples of nominal data. The labelling could be reversed or swapped around without loss of information. We are not suggesting that males are ahead of females (or *vice versa*) or that one locality is ordered ahead of another. The labels are just for our convenience, perhaps for data entry. We could have used letters or Roman numerals instead without any forfeit.

For ordinal data, the order is important. So, for question 1 in the examples in section 4.7, the answers are ordinal in nature, rising from 'none' to 'very mild' to 'mild' to 'moderate' to 'severe' to 'very severe'. They could just as easily have been labelled in the reverse order, from 'very severe' down to 'none', but they are ordered. The important point to make is that, while there is order in the options, we are not saying anything about the relative differences between options. We cannot say, for example, that the difference between 'mild' and 'very mild' is the same as that between 'mild' and 'moderate'. Furthermore, although 'moderate' is labelled '4' and 'very mild' is labelled '2' in this instance, we cannot say that moderate pain is twice as severe as that of very mild pain. The Likert scale is an ordinal scale: e.g. from strongly disagree to strongly agree.

Another type of data is **discrete data**. Discrete data increases in steps. So, a count of people would increase in steps of 1: 1, 2, 3, 4 .... You cannot have 1.5 or 2.3 or 11.9 people. Finally, there is **continuous data**, for which it is possible to get any point in between two numbers. So, even if we record the length of a piece of string to the nearest centimetre, the length of the string could actually be 1.1223 cm or 0.786772 cm or any other number between 0.5 cm and 1.5 cm if it was recorded as 1 cm.

Continuous and discrete data can be split into interval and ratio measured scales. **Interval scales** are reasonably rare and the normal example given is that of temperature in degrees Celsius. The difference between 35°C and 40°C is the same as that between 30°C and 35°C. Similarly, the difference between 30 cm and 40 cm is the same as that between 10 cm and 20 cm. However, interval scales, unlike ratio scales, do not have a meaningful zero point. 0°C does not mean there is no temperature, it just indicates the freezing point of water. Similarly, we cannot say that 40°C is twice as hot as 20°C. However, we can say that a piece of string measuring 40 cm is twice as long as one measuring 20 cm; and this is a **ratio scale**. 0 cm means there is no length. There is no meaningful zero point on an interval scale; values can be added and subtracted but not multiplied or divided, which they can be if they are measured on a ratio scale. Do not worry too much about the difference between interval and ratio scales. As long as you can distinguish them from nominal and ordinal scales then that is the main thing.

Often, what are theoretically ordinal scales are interpreted as interval scales to allow more common types of analysis to be performed.

This is particularly true where the respondent is asked to give a rating. For example, patients are asked to rate their happiness with an explanation they have been given about their treatment, on a scale of 1–10. Our view is that it is still an ordinal scale and it is subjective as to whether it can be treated as an interval scale. Such scales are often analysed as interval scales but, although the end result will often not be too dissimilar, we would err on the side of caution and treat them as ordinal scales. The main reason why ordinal scales like these are often treated as interval scales is because the method of analysis is different depending on the type of measurement scale assumed and interval/ratio scale analyses tend to be the more common and, therefore, the better known. However, this is no reason to risk using the wrong analysis and obtaining the wrong outcomes. The different analyses may well give similar results and if you are unsure whether the measurement scale can be classified as at least interval, it is best to use ordinal methods of analysis.

5.6 AIMS OF ANALYSIS

The aims of an analysis could be varied but there are a number of common aspects to analysis of different studies and these include the following.

- **Summarizing the characteristics of the study population**; for example, in our LLI study it could be the proportion of people with an LLI or the mean scores on the health profile SF-36 scales; or in the hospital satisfaction study it could be the overall level of satisfaction of people's stay in hospital.

- **Indicating how widely individuals differ.** We know people will give different answers to the same questions. A mean score on an SF-36 scale does not indicate that everybody scored around this average: many may have scored much higher or much lower. Not everybody will have the same amount of satisfaction with their stay in hospital.

- **Showing relationships between variables**: are mental health scores related to physical health scores? Do the older age groups or people in different socioeconomic categories tend to be more (or less) satisfied with hospital stays? Notice, in this last idea we are returning to the idea of dependent and independent variables, which we touched on earlier.

- Closely related to the last aim is the idea of **describing differences between sections of the study population**; for example, differences between people reporting an LLI and those who do not or the survival patterns and quality of life between a group of patients given one treatment for a disease compared to another group with the same disease but a different treatment.

In all these aims, we should be thinking about what we can **infer** from our data about the study population from which we drew the sample. This takes us into the realms of **inferential** statistics. We shall meet these later but we need to start simply and work our way to more complicated techniques, if needed.

Again, we must highlight the necessity to concentrate on your starting hypotheses and the aims of the study, and not to allow yourself to be side-tracked down side alleys and get lost in your data.

5.7 INITIAL DATA INSPECTION

5.7.1 Introduction to descriptive analysis

The statement at the end of this paragraph may bring good cheer or disappointment to you depending on whether you are a little afraid (or, perhaps, wary) of getting too far down the statistical track or whether you are eager to jump into the more exciting realms of statistical inference. The fact is that you should start any analysis by simply describing the data. What does the data tell you about your sample? The rest of this chapter covers description of data by use of graphs and tables. The next chapter is concerned with use of averages and other numbers to summarize interval and ratio-scaled data. It is only in Chapter 7 that we shall start thinking about relating our sample data to the study population as a whole and about inferences concerning the population based on what we know about the sample. In other words, we shall move from **descriptive** statistics into the (supposedly more glamorous) world of **inferential** statistics. And now for that statement we promised you: the amount and importance of the inferential analysis we do depends very much on our descriptive analysis and the objectives of our study. This will hopefully become clear as we move along through the murky undergrowth of descriptive statistics.

For example, we found that 33% of our sample reported an LLI. Later we shall consider the issues around saying that such a figure might be representative of a larger population.

5.7.2 Tables and graphs

The most common and attractive way of summarizing and presenting data is in the form of tables or graphs. These provide a quick way of displaying data and allow breaks to be made in solid rows of turgid text. However, both tables and graphs can be produced well and informatively, without lies or leading to misconceptions, or they can be done badly. Both Huff (1973) and Tufte (1983) display graphs that have been published in leading and respected journals and newspapers, some elaborately produced, which are misleading, impossible to interpret or simply give the impression the creator wanted to give, whether the data backs this up or not. Both of these texts we can recommend as light reading on how to, and how not to, produce graphs (the book by Huff also explores other misuses of statistics).

Both tables and graphs should have basic characteristics. It should be stated here that most statistical software packages leave a lot to be desired in their production of tables and graphs. Remember, these packages tend to give standard formats for their tables and graphs, which may not be suitable for your data and purposes. You may have to make extensive use of the 'options' procedures to make them more user-friendly and informative, or redesign or edit them yourself.

The main thing to remember is that the table (or graph) should be able to tell the story (the correct story) without reference to the text. Include a title so that the reader knows what the table or graph is about. Label both axes of the graph (with units of measurement, if necessary, e.g. centimetres or pounds sterling). Label the rows and columns of the table likewise, and give the row and column totals or percentages where they would be useful. Do not clutter the table or graph so it becomes difficult to read. Be careful about squashing the axes or scales of a graph. Removing the origin can lead to misleading charts. Above all, think of the visual presentation of the graph: does it suggest the truth or is it in anyway misleading or exaggerating the truth?

5.8 NOMINAL AND ORDINAL DATA

5.8.1 Frequency distributions

We shall start off by considering table presentations for categorical data and by looking at frequency distributions. There are many words that seem to arise time and again in statistics (as in every subject, one would suspect). The word **distribution** is very important and one of the basics of statistics is to assess the distribution of data. One of the ways to do it with this type of measurement of data is by frequency distributions. A distribution shows the values of variables, from lowest to highest value, across the units (for example, people) under investigation.

A **frequency distribution** is simply all the possible values for a variable together with their frequencies (i.e. a count of all occurrences of that value). Associated with this is the **relative frequency**, which is the proportion of all observations (or respondents in a sample survey) that have that particular value. This is simply a percentage (%) and is calculated as follows:

$$\frac{\text{no. of units with that value}}{\text{total no. of units}} \times 100$$

Let us give a simple example of this and consider the first question on the SF-36 and the number of people who reported an LLI in the first stage. The frequencies together with relative frequencies are shown in Tables 5.2 and 5.3.

These are simple tables but they are descriptive without further comment needed. However, we reserve our right to now comment further! Notice the obligatory title, which also explains the tables and the

Table 5.2

Frequency table for question 'How do you rate your health in general?'

Rating	No. of people	%
Excellent	91	7.6
Very good	293	24.6
Good	410	34.4
Fair	308	25.8
Poor	91	7.6
Total	1193	100

headings for the columns. Table 5.2 has an ordinal scale from 'Excellent' down to 'Poor'. A total of 91 people answered 'Excellent' and this works out as 7.6% of those who answered. This is calculated as (91 / 1193) × 100. The total percentage comes to 100%, as it should do (reliant on rounding errors) as all the respondents are included in the table.

Table 5.3

Results of survey into limiting long-term illness

Reported LLI?	No. of people	%
Yes	947	33.0
No	1920	67.0
Total	2867	100

Relative frequencies are tied up with probability. A probability of 1 is equivalent to a 100% chance. A probability of 0 is equivalent to a 0% chance. In the example above in Table 5.2, if we selected one person at random from the people included in the table, we would have a 7.6% chance, or probability of 0.076 (7.6 divided by 100), of selecting someone who stated that their health was 'Excellent'. This is quite a small probability. Another way of looking at it is that just under 8 in every 100 people answered 'Excellent' to the question.

Let us now consider how the original table looked using the SPSS for Windows output (Table 5.4; we have cleaned it up here).

Table 5.4

Frequency distribution as produced by SPSS for Windows

SF1 GH general

Value Label	Value	Frequency	Percent	Valid Percent	Cum Percent
Excellent	1	91	7.6	7.6	7.6
Very good	2	293	24.3	24.6	32.2
Good	3	409	33.9	34.3	66.5
Fair	4	308	25.6	25.8	92.3
Poor	5	91	7.6	7.6	99.9
	33	1	0.1	0.1	100.0
	9	12	1.0	Missing	
	Total	1205	100.0	100.0	

Valid cases   1193   Missing cases   12

As you can see Table 5.4 is a little more complicated than our table. This table needs extra scrutiny. Each of the five options in Table 5.2 is included together with their code (or 'value' as SPSS calls it). However, we have two extra categories. We have a category with no label but with the value '33'. This is puzzling as there should be no-one with a value 33 for this question since the values for this question run from 1–5. Reference back to the spreadsheet and back to that person's questionnaire reveals a typing error: this person really answered 'Good' or value 3, so we can correct this, as has been done in Table 5.2. The missing row (value 9) shows the number of people who left this question blank (or, perhaps, gave an improper answer such as circling more than one option), and this accounts for 12 people whom we remove from the analysis. Remember, we defined '9.0' as a missing value earlier so it would not be included in the analysis. Therefore, the figures we want for relative frequencies are under the column headed 'Valid Percent' (once we have corrected the typing error). 'Cum Percent' is the cumulative percentage. So, for example, 32.2% answered either 'Excellent' or 'Very good', the percentage figure relating to those who answered 'Excellent' added to the percentage figure relating to those who answered 'Very good'.

5.8.2 Cross-tabulations

Let's explore a bit more. Table 5.3 tells us that 33% of people who responded to our survey reported having an LLI. If we selected one person at random from the respondents to our survey, we would have a probability of 0.33 that they would have reported an LLI; alternatively we would have a probability of (1 − 0.33) or 0.67 that they reported no LLI.

This information is great as far as it goes, but a lot more information than this can be obtained. Let's break Table 5.3 down a bit further and look at the rates based on age and sex categories in a cross-tabulation (Table 5.5).

Age–sex category	No. reporting LLI (%)	No. reporting no LLI (%)	Total
18–44			
Male	55 (11)	441 (89)	496
Female	60 (11)	488 (89)	548
45–64			
Male	200 (37)	340 (63)	540
Female	198 (32)	421 (68)	619
65–74			
Male	119 (58)	86 (42)	205
Female	155 (62)	73 (38)	228
75+			
Male	51 (66)	26 (34)	77
Female	109 (71)	45 (29)	154
Total	947	1920	2867

Table 5.5

Prevalence of LLI broken down by age and sex

Now, that is a bit more informative. The percentages go across the rows and the totals in the end column are those for the individual rows. The bottom row gives the totals for the individual columns. Look how the rates for LLI increase as the age groups get older. Only around one in every 10 people between 18 years and 44 years reported an LLI, but this figure increases dramatically and around two people in every three reported an LLI in the 75 and over age group. We do not think, as we have a good sample size, that we need any analytical techniques to demonstrate that, for our population at least, rates of LLI increase with age. This illustrates the benefit of a descriptive analysis first of all before troubling ourselves with any inferential analysis techniques. We might, however, wish to assess whether males are more or less likely to report an LLI than females. The differences vary depending on age group. This is something we could do using techniques that will be described in Chapter 10. Obviously there is no one right way to produce a table, and perhaps you would like to redesign this table to see if you can improve on it, taking into account the features we stated previously that are desirable in a table.

Including both the numbers and the percentages gives more information. Just giving a percentage (such as 25%) does not indicate from how many this comes – it could be four or 400 000 – while just giving the numbers normally makes it harder for readers to compare data across groups or populations.

We have actually jumped from one variable to three variables in Table 5.5; reporting of LLI or not, age and sex. We could have produced a table of age by prevalence of LLI, or sex by prevalence of LLI if we had wanted to.

Notice that in this example we have collapsed a continuous variable (age) into a categorical variable based on age ranges. We could have produced one row for each age value but this would probably have left us with about 60 or 70 rows, littered with cell counts of 0, 1 and 2. Instead of that, we decided on sensible groupings, which are similar to those used in other surveys such as the Census.

We are now really at the limit of the amount of information we can get into a table, certainly in terms of number of variables, without making the table confusing, difficult to read and cluttered. Computer packages will give you many options as to what information you wish to have recorded in your table. As an experiment, we produced a simple cross-tabulation (or crosstabs for short) of age group against reporting of an LLI or not and checked the boxes of some of the options for inclusion in the table in SPSS for Windows (we could have checked three more!). Table 5.6 shows the mass of figures.

At first site it looks a jumble of figures and does not make for easy reading (hint: do not crowd tables for presentation like this!). The top left-hand corner is your guide to what is going on, so the top figure in each cell (or part of the table) is simply the count, or observed value (e.g. 66 people aged 18–44 answered the question 'Very good'). The next figure down is the expected value ('Exp Val') based on the data. Do not worry about this for the time being: we shall come back to this in Chapter 10. It refers to what is the expected value in each cell of the table based on the row and column totals. The third figure down is the row percentage. So, 36.3% of 18–44-year-olds answered 'Very good'. The fourth figure is the column percentage; 22.5% of those who answered 'Very good' were in the 18–44-year age group. The bottom figure is the total percentage, so 5.5% of all the respondents answered 'Very good' and were aged between 18 and 44. We can also see that

Table 5.6

Example of SPSS for Windows output for age against answers for SF-36 question 1

AGE GROUP	Age group by SF1	GH	general			
		SF1				
Count Exp Val Row Pct Col Pct Tot Pct	Excellent	Very good	Good	Fair	Poor	Row Total
	1	2	3	4	5	
AGE GROUP						
1	29	66	55	24	8	182
18–44	13.9	44.7	62.5	47.0	13.9	15.3%
	15.9%	36.3%	30.2%	13.2%	4.4%	
	31.9%	22.5%	13.4%	7.8%	8.8%	
	2.4%	5.5%	4.6%	2.0%	0.7%	
2	49	151	198	136	35	569
45–64	43.4	139.7	195.5	146.9	43.4	47.7%
	8.6%	26.5%	34.8%	23.9%	6.2%	
	53.8%	51.5%	48.3%	44.2%	38.5%	
	4.1%	12.7%	16.6%	11.4%	2.9%	
3	11	57	107	93	18	286
65–74	21.8	70.2	98.3	73.8	21.8	24.0%
	3.8%	19.9%	37.4%	32.5%	6.3%	
	12.1%	19.5%	26.1%	30.2%	19.8%	
	0.9%	4.8%	9.0%	7.8%	1.5%	
4	2	19	50	55	30	156
75+	11.9	38.3	53.6	40.3	11.9	13.1%
	1.3%	12.2%	32.1%	35.3%	19.2%	
	2.2%	6.5%	12.2%	17.9%	33.0%	
	0.2%	1.6%	4.2%	4.6%	2.5%	
Column Total	91 7.6%	293 24.6%	410 34.4%	308 25.8%	91 7.6%	1193 100.0%

Number of Missing Observations: 12

15.3% of respondents were aged between 18 and 44 and, as seen before, 24.6% answered 'Very good'.

It is up to you, the user, to decide which are the key figures to include (certainly the count and the row and column totals, as well as a percentage; in this case, probably the row percentage is most informative).

One final table example will suffice for now, taken this time from the hospital satisfaction survey. This gives an example where percentages are not really needed, certainly with small sample sizes like the one in Table 5.7.

Percentages can be superfluous and proportions can be easier to read. So, in Table 5.7, 11 out of 24 (11 / 24) females stated they thought the care they received was excellent, compared to 14 / 25 males, and 19 / 24 females thought their care was excellent or very good compared to 23 / 25 males.

Table 5.7

Answers to question 'Overall, how would you rate the care you received at this hospital?'

	Female	Male	Total
Excellent	11	14	25
Very good	8	9	17
Good	3	1	4
Fair	1	1	2
Poor	1	0	1
Total	24	25	49

NB: 1 female did not answer the question

5.8.3 Graphical representations of nominal/ordinal data

Let us now consider how we could represent some of our data graphically. There are two common types of graph used for representing categorical data. We will consider the data in Table 5.2 first and construct a **pie-chart** for this data (Figure 5.2).

Figure 5.2

Pie chart for question 'How do you rate your health in general?'

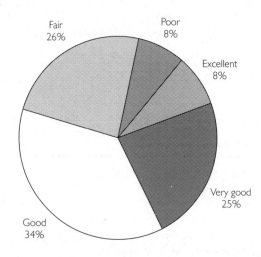

A pie-chart is a circle divided into segments with each segment representing the relative proportion for each category. For example, 'Excellent' accounts for 7.6% of the answers from the study population and therefore takes up 7.6% of the area of the circle. There are 360 degrees in a circle so the method of calculation is as follows:

$$\frac{\text{no. of units with that value}}{\text{total no. of units}} \times 360$$

This, then, is the angle taken by that category in the centre of the pie-chart. The total value for all the angles will add up to 360.

It is noticeable that there will normally be less data shown in a graph and that is why a lot of people prefer tables even though graphs can normally quickly highlight interesting features. However, notice that the pie-chart does not detail how many people were in each category or how big the sample was – it could have been 15 or 10 000.

Figure 5.3 displays **bar charts** representing the data in the pie-chart.

Figure 5.3a shows the same data as Figure 5.2 except that this time you can see the frequencies rather than the percentages. The categories are labelled at the bottom and the frequencies up the side. The gaps between the columns show that the data is categorical: i.e. the groupings are distinct, there is a clear cut off point between the categories.

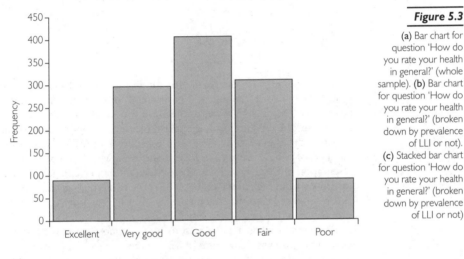

(a)

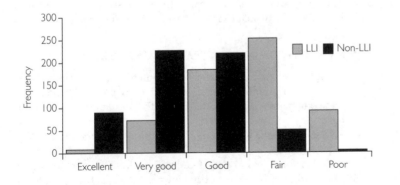

(b)

Figure 5.3

(a) Bar chart for question 'How do you rate your health in general?' (whole sample). (b) Bar chart for question 'How do you rate your health in general?' (broken down by prevalence of LLI or not). (c) Stacked bar chart for question 'How do you rate your health in general?' (broken down by prevalence of LLI or not)

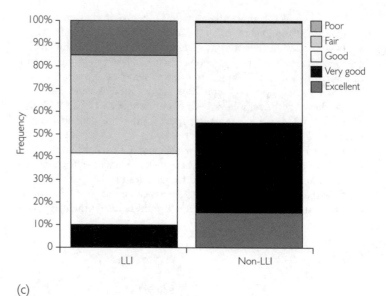

(c)

Figure 5.3b compares the results for the LLI group and the non-LLI group. As expected, the non-LLI group tend to see their health more favourably. Figure 5.3b works as there are very similar numbers in the two groups, LLI and non-LLI. If one had been appreciably smaller than the other the graph could have been misleading in terms of the relative numbers of people in each category. Figure 5.3c would be a better representation of the data: we get a better idea of the percentages in each category within each of the groups. Here, the two groups get a bar each and it is 'stacked' so that the percentage in each category covers that proportion of the height of the bar.

We could extend Figure 5.3b to more groups, perhaps breaking down the two groups by sex to have four columns for each category. This, however, would start making the graph difficult to read and giving it the appearance of being cluttered. Remember, the graph should be clear and easy to read. Bar charts are often displayed horizontally as well as vertically (which is how they are arranged in Figure 5.3).

5.9 GRAPHS FOR INTERVAL/RATIO SCALE DATA

The graphs in this section are those that tend to be used for interval and ratio scale data. Another type of graph, the boxplot, will be looked at in the next chapter where we shall also discuss summarizing this type of data.

We start with the **histogram**. Example histograms are shown in Figures 5.4 and 5.5.

These are for two of the SF-36 scales; Physical Functioning (PF) and General Health (GH). Notice how the non-LLI group have higher numbers of people at the highest end of the scale, i.e. towards the best

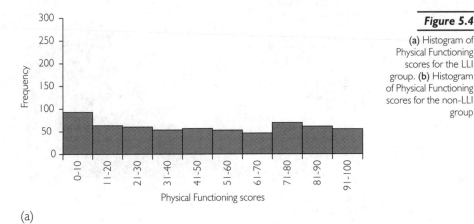

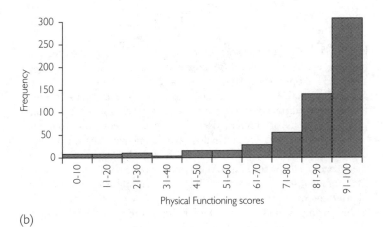

(a)

(b)

Figure 5.4

(a) Histogram of Physical Functioning scores for the LLI group. (b) Histogram of Physical Functioning scores for the non-LLI group

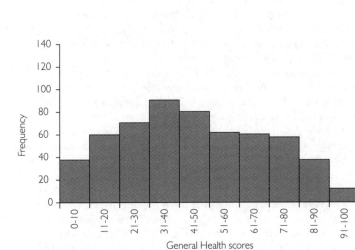

(a)

Figure 5.5

(a) Histogram of General Health scores for the LLI group. (b) Histogram of General Health scores for the non-LLI group

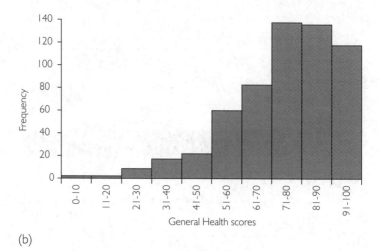

(b)

health. The different values are on the horizontal (*x*) axis and their frequencies are on the vertical (*y*) axis. As you can see, we have categorized the continuous variable but, as the variable is continuous, there are no gaps between the bars. On a bar-chart there are gaps between the bars to indicate a distinction between categories but histograms display continuous or discrete data that logically flow on from one another. Histograms are normally vertical and you should be concerned not only with the height of the bars in the histogram but also the area taken up by the bars. If the widths of the bars are identical then the heights of the bars represent the frequencies. However, it is possible to draw histograms with different widths (which must be the case if the groupings used are of different sizes on the horizontal axis). In this case, the area is proportional to the frequency.

Notice that we have kept the scale of the *y*-axis the same for the LLI and the non-LLI graphs, i.e. going up to a frequency of 320 for Physical Functioning and 140 for General Health. This gives a better comparison when the sample sizes are similar, as in this case.

The histogram is a useful method of assessing the **distribution** of interval/ratio data. As can be seen from the histograms of Physical Functioning and General Health, the data for the non-LLI group is skewed much more towards the healthier scores, i.e. higher frequencies near the 100 (best health) end. We shall return to this idea of representing distributions by the use of histograms in the next chapter.

Interval and ratio data can be represented graphically in a number of other ways including line-graphs, stem and leaf plots and scatterplots.

The **stem and leaf plot** in Figure 5.6 represents the General Health score of people aged between 18 and 64 with a self-reported LLI.

The stem gives the first number of the age (i.e. the tens – 0, 10, 20, 30, 40, etc.) and the numbers to the right are the units. Hence, the first five people score 0, the next five people score 5 and the next eight score

0	0000055555
I	0000000005555555555555555
2	000000000000000000055555555555555555555555555
3	00000000000000235555555555555555555555555555555577777777
4	000000000000000000022222225555555555555777777777
5	000000002222222222255557777777777
6	022222222222222222225777777777777777779
7	2222222222222222222222777777777778
8	02222222222222222277777777
9	2222777
I0	00

Figure 5.6

A stem and leaf plot of General Health for the LLI group, aged 18–64

10. Each number to the right of the line represents one case (or person) – although this is not always true, it can represent more than one case for big sample sizes. Again, we can see that this is a way of representing the distribution of the data and gives the same idea of the shape of the distribution as a histogram. This is a much more symmetrical distribution.

The **scatterplot** is a method of representing two variables (or bivariate data) and is shown in Figure 5.7.

For each case (person in this example from the LLI survey) the first variable is plotted against the second variable. Here we have plotted Physical Functioning (PF) score against General Health (GH) score. As you can see from Figure 5.7, the values for PF, as expected, tend to increase as the values for GH increase. This is another way of identifying outliers and errors. The case numbered '337' could be considered an outlier (maybe an error: we would go away and check the values for this person). Scatterplots are also very useful for looking at associations between different variables as we shall see when we look at correlation and regression later on.

A final graph which can be useful is the **line-graph**, this is particularly useful in plotting changes over time. Figure 5.8a is (a fictional) account of the GH score on the SF-36 taken at regular intervals from someone obtaining regular treatment.

Just to show how graphs can be 'manipulated', compare it with Figure 5.8b and notice the different impressions they leave on you. It is, of course, the same data plotted on a different scale. We have been naughty by starting at 45 and ending at 75 in Figure 5.8b and have also

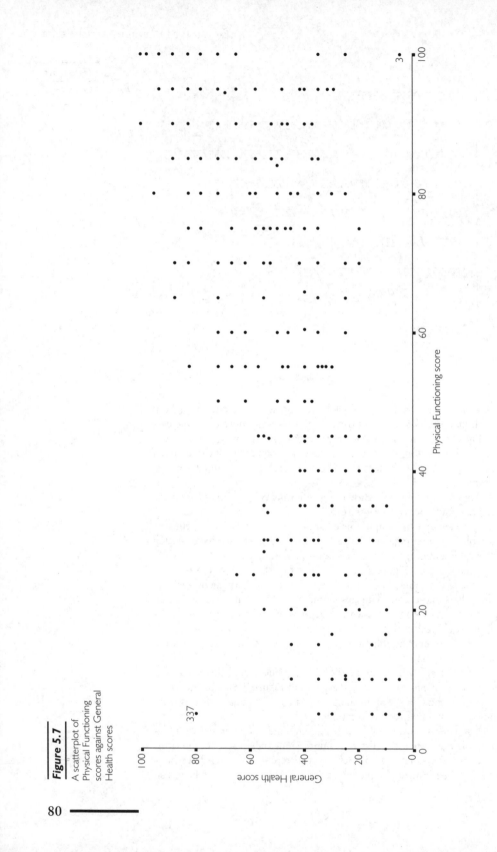

Figure 5.7

A scatterplot of Physical Functioning scores against General Health scores

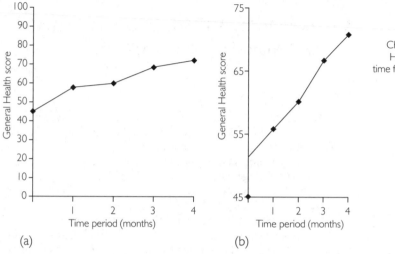

**Figure 5.8
(a & b)**

Change in General
Health score over
time for one individual

(a)   (b)

squashed the *x*-axis. Figure 5.8a gives the better impression of the improvement, giving the whole range of possible scores from 0 to 100.

5.10 SUMMARY

We have learned in this chapter how to get started in our data analysis and how to think about presenting data accurately and attractively. You can always make graphs more attractive by using different colours and shading of bars but, remember, it is the visual interpretation and the self-explanatory quality that are needed in graphs and tables. Do they tell the truth?

Although graphs are more visually appealing, more information can be presented in a table and they are less susceptible to 'manipulation'.

In the next chapter we look at descriptive techniques for summarizing interval and ratio data and the important idea of the normal distribution. The ideas and techniques learnt in this and the next chapter, while not going into great statistical complexity, are the basis for the rest of the text and, because of this, may be the most important chapters in the book.

6 Averages, measures of spread and the normal distribution

6.1 Introduction

'Average' is a general word that is often meant to indicate something quite specific. There is the 'law of averages', there are batting averages in cricket and baseball, there are the averages loved by newspaper and magazine contributors and companies in advertising their services and products. 'The average family has 2.4 children, one car and two pets'; 'the average lifetime of our battery is over 20% longer than our nearest rival'.

Complications arise from the fact that there are a number of measures of average that could be used, and often the reader is left to guess which one has been used. We shall concentrate on the three that appear most frequently: the **arithmetic mean**, the **median** and the **mode**.

If you went to the doctor with a particular illness and the doctor said that, on average, the illness would clear up on its own after 14 days, you might start getting worried if you were still ill after 17 days. However, if you knew in actual fact that 80% of people recovered in between 13 and 21 days you would not be so worried. Therefore, as well as a measure of average (or **centrality**) it is necessary to give some idea of the extent to which the data is spread out around the middle point, its variability in other words, and this will form the second part of this chapter.

Finally, the way in which this spread of values is patterned (the distribution) plays a very important part in statistics and we already have commented on this in the previous chapter. We shall end this chapter by looking at distributions in more detail.

Remember that we have taken a sample from a population (known as the study population) to obtain information about that population. We are using the sample statistic to estimate the population statistic (e.g. mean, median or variance). If we had information about everyone in the population then we could calculate the population statistic; otherwise we calculate the sample statistic and use this as an estimate for the population statistic. The calculations we are performing in sections 6.2 to 6.4 are identical for both the population and the sample statistic except that we use the population size (number of people in the population) for the population statistic and the sample size (number of people for which we actually have a value for the variable being investigated) for the sample statistic. The one exception to this is the variance (and, hence, the standard deviation), which we shall explain shortly.

6.2 THE MEAN, THE MEDIAN AND THE MODE

On mentioning the word 'average', most people assume this to indicate the mean, and by stating the mean, they assume it is the arithmetic mean. In the majority of cases this is usually what people are implying, or assuming others will take for granted; they calculate a mean and state it as 'the average'. Just to make things even more complicated there is actually more than one type of mean, but the word 'mean' is most closely associated with the arithmetic mean and if anything else is used it is usually stated in full (e.g. the 'geometric mean' or the even rarer 'harmonic mean'). Therefore, when we talk about 'the mean' in this text, we are referring to the arithmetic mean.

6.2.1 Definitions

The mean and median are most appropriately used for interval and ratio data. They have been used for ordinal data as well but care needs to be taken over the interpretation and the appropriateness of these measures for ordinal data. As a general rule, means and medians should only be used for interval and ratio data, i.e. non-categorical data. The mode is less commonly used and, as will be seen, is a way of expressing the value with the highest frequency, making it more useful for categorical data.

We shall now give some definitions and hope a couple of examples will suffice to clarify the differences between these measures and when it is best to use each.

- **Arithmetic mean:** 'the sum of the values divided by the number of values', the population mean is often denoted by μ and the sample mean by either $\hat{\mu}$ or $\bar{x}$.
- **Median:** 'the middle value when all the values are arranged in order'.
- **Mode:** 'the most frequently occurring value'.

6.2.2 Examples of calculating the mean, median and mode

Although you are most likely to use computers to calculate these statistics, it is important to understand the principles of what is going on. Later, we shall explore a printout of a SPSS for Windows output summary including mean, median and mode as well as a host of other statistics. But, for now, a simple example using Figure 5.1 and the first 10 records and their corresponding value for the variable 'age' will get us under way. Let us imagine that these 10 people represent a sample of people from a larger population. These values for age are shown below:

36 39 40 20 67 18 29 20 72 50

In order to calculate the median, and to make it easier to find the mode, we need to arrange these values in order of size. This is done in Table 6.1, and the values for the three measures of average are highlighted.

Table 6.1	72	
Calculating the three measures of average	67	
	50	
	40	
	39	
		* middle score (median) = 37.5
	36	
	29	
	20	
		* most common score (mode) = 20
	20	
	18	
	—	
	391	* 391 divided by 10 = 39.1 (mean)

The mean is calculated using the sum of all the values (72 + 67 + ... + 18), which equals 391. There are 10 values so the mean is simply 391 divided by 10, which equals 39.1. It is normal to write the population size as N and the sample size as n. The calculation for the population mean is the same as for the sample mean except, obviously, n is replaced by N (the sample size by the population size).

The sample size is the number of people for whom we actually have the information (i.e. the variable measurements). If we had 11 people in our above example but one had not given us their age we would have used 10 in the calculation as we have 10 ages.

To calculate the median, you add 1 to the number of values and divide by 2 to find the midpoint (i.e. $(n + 1) / 2$ where n is the number of values). The midpoint here, therefore, is $(10 + 1) / 2$ which equals 5.5. The midpoint is, therefore, half way between the fifth and sixth values (i.e. $(39 + 36) / 2$), which equals 37.5. If we had 11 values instead of 10, the median would be the sixth value $((11 + 1) / 2)$.

The mode is 20, as this occurs twice and other values only occur once each. On this occasion, the mode is not particularly useful: it does not say much about the data. If one of the other values had occurred twice as well, we would have had a distribution with two modal points, which is called **bimodal.**

The mean and median are very similar and both reflect the data pretty well (although we still need the measures of spread, which will be discussed shortly). However, suppose that there had been a typing mistake and that the oldest person's age was entered as 172 rather than the correct figure of 72. The mean immediately leaps to 491 / 10 = 49.1. There are now only three people older than the mean. The median remains at 37.5: it is not affected by extreme values; indeed, it does not matter what the values are on either side of the midpoint. The mean, though, is affected by extreme values, the so-called 'outliers'. If we got this result in our analysis, we would go back and check our data and observe and correct the mistake (if we had not already discovered it through the techniques described in the last chapter). However, what if the figure for the oldest person had been 121 (the age of the oldest living person at the time of writing)? This is a plausible (though unlikely) age and might just be an outlier rather than an error. We would need to check carefully that this was, indeed, a true value. The mean has risen to 44.0 thanks to the effect of this outlier.

If the figure of 121 is accurate, then the median gives us more accurate information about the data. It is less misleading even though it does not use as much information as the mean. Therefore, when calculating or displaying means, we need to check on outliers or skewed information (i.e. where more figures are found towards the end of the ranges, towards either the largest or the smallest values). We shall look more closely at what are known as **skewed distributions** and the occasions when it is best to use the mean or median later.

Another way of eliminating outliers or extreme values but using most of the data is by use of the trimmed mean. This is used when outliers (or extreme observations) are suspected. A 5% trimmed mean tells us that the smallest 5% of values and the largest 5% have been removed and the mean calculated based on the remaining 90% of values. This is sometimes preferred to the median when extreme values are suspected because it makes use of more of the data than the median but, like the median, should be less influenced by outlying observations.

The mode's usefulness in summarizing interval and ratio data has often been derided. It is more valid, perhaps, when looking at categorical-type data. For example, if a doctor stated that the average hip replacement was performed on females aged over 65 then this would be an example of using the mode. The most often occurring recipient of a hip replacement is female, over the age of 65.

6.3 VARIABILITY

Consider the following two distributions:

```
1)  99  100  100  100  101
2)   0   50  100  150  200
```

Both of these have identical means (and medians) of 100 (please check!) but their distributions are clearly different. One ranges from 99–101, the other from 0–200. Identifying the mean and median on their own might give us the impression that the data sets were identical (or at least, very similar) when, in reality, they are very different, with one having a much wider spread of values than the other. Some idea of the extent of spread or **variability** in the data sets is needed.

6.3.1 Variance and standard deviation

If you are going to report a mean, you must either report the standard deviation (SD) or a confidence interval for the mean (we shall look at confidence intervals in the next chapter). Any self-respecting journal would not accept papers reporting means alone and you should get suspicious if you read a paper that only gives the mean because the mean cannot tell the whole story.

A couple of definitions:

- 'The variance is the mean of the squared differences between each individual observation and the overall mean of these observations'.
- 'The standard deviation is the square root of the variance'.

The standard deviation is, in effect, the average deviation from the mean of the observed values. The rather clumsy way of reaching the standard deviation (squaring the differences to get a variance, then taking the square root) is a way of making the value of the standard deviation always positive (or zero). If the values are spread out, then they will be both greater and smaller than the mean. A zero value indicates that all the values are the same as the mean; as the spread of data increases, so the value of the standard deviation will increase.

Shortly, we will look at what you can say about the distribution of your data by looking at the standard deviation. Firstly, though, let us look at how they are calculated (skip this section out if you are beginning to feel mathematically challenged).

If we had information on the variable we were investigating for everyone in the population we would calculate the **population variance** (σ^2). If we have taken a sample, we must estimate the population variance by calculating the sample variance (s^2).

In a population there are N values. Each value is taken in turn and the mean value for the whole population is subtracted from it and the result squared. The results (N of them) are then summed and divided by N.

Going back to our example of 6.2.2, we can now calculate the variance and standard deviation, assuming here that these 10 values are from the 10 people who make up the whole population we are studying (they obviously do not, but let us imagine they do for the moment). $N = 10$, and the population mean $\mu = 39.1$

$$(72 - 39.1)^2 + (67 - 39.1)^2 + (50 - 39.1)^2 + (40 - 39.1)^2 + (39 - 39.1)^2 + (36 - 39.1)^2 + (29 - 39.1)^2 + (20 - 39.1)^2 + (20 - 39.1)^2 + (18 - 39.1)^2 = 3266.9$$

Then divide this by the population size, 10. The variance (σ^2) is 3266.9 / 10, which equals 326.69. The standard deviation (σ) is the square root of this, which is $\sqrt{326.69} = 18.07$.

Now let us go back to our original example where these 10 people are a sample from the population we are studying. We do not have information about everyone in the population – only about those in our sample. For the **sample variance** (s^2) we replace N by $n - 1$, where n is the sample size. We deduct one as this gives a more unbiased estimate of the population variance, although the larger the sample size the less effect it has on the figures for the variance and standard deviation. For more detail on why this is so, see, for example, Clarke and Cooke (1992).

So, for the sample variance we have: 3266.9 / 9 = 362.99 and the standard deviation, s, is $\sqrt{362.99}$ which is 19.05. Note how this has increased because we are now only **estimating** the population variance from our sample data.

For small samples of data, a suitable calculator can be used to derive standard deviations, and you will find that they offer the choice of a population standard deviation or a sample standard deviation.

The variance is measured in the square of the original units of the data; so, if we had calculated the mean length of a piece of string in centimetres (cm), the variance would be in the form of centimetres squared (cm^2). The standard deviation is measured in the original units, so, like the mean, in this case it would be measured in centimetres. The units of the original measurement should be reported whichever measure of average and spread you are using.

6.3.2 Percentiles and quartiles

Measures of spread for the median tend to have fewer mathematical formulae. They are based on **percentiles**. The kth percentile is the value below which k% of the values fall when arranged in ascending order. Hence, the median is the 50th percentile, since 50% of the values fall below it. Common percentile values are the 10th (indicating that the lowest 10% of values fall below it), 25th (known as the lower quartile and indicating the lowest quarter of values fall below it), the 50th (the median), the 75th (the **upper quartile**; three-quarters of the values fall below this value) and the 90th (just the largest 10% of values will be above this value). Or you may see work based on quintiles, which divide the data into fifths, i.e. the 20th, 40th, 60th and 80th percentiles. The range between the lower and upper quartiles is known as the **interquartile** range and half of this range is the semi-interquartile range. Often when the median is reported you will get what is known as the **five number summary**, namely:

- the minimum value;
- the lower quartile;
- the median;
- the upper quartile;
- the maximum value.

The range of the values is the distance between the minimum and the maximum values.

If we now go back to the data in section 6.2.2, the five number summary of the data can be calculated (Table 6.2):

The upper quartile can be most easily calculated by finding the median of all the numbers above the median value, i.e. ignoring the median value and all the values below it. Similarly, the lower quartile can be calculated by finding the median of all the numbers below the median value.

Many medical journals now advise the presentation of the interquartile range whenever the median is used to summarize data.

Table 6.2		
Calculating the five number summary of data	72	* maximum = 72
	67	
	50	* upper quartile = 50
	40	
	39	
		* median = 37.5
	36	
	29	
	20	* lower quartile = 20
	20	
	18	* minimum = 18
	Range = (18, 72)	
	Interquartile range = (20, 50)	

It is possible to represent this five figure summary in the form of a chart, known as a **boxplot**, and two are shown in Figure 6.1.

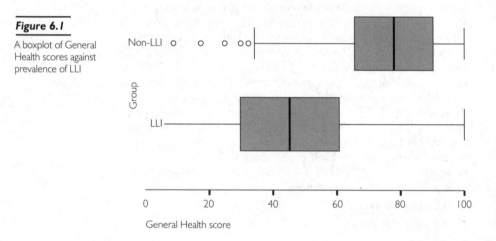

Figure 6.1

A boxplot of General Health scores against prevalence of LLI

This figure compares the General Health (GH) scale scores from the SF-36 for the LLI group (the bottom plot) against the non-LLI group (the top plot). The box starts at the lower quartile value and ends at the upper quartile value. The line in the box represents the median. The lines from the box stretch to the minimum and maximum values; however, SPSS for Windows defines 'outliers' and 'extreme values' differently. A value is considered an outlier if it is between 1.5 and 3 times the length of the box away from the box. The circles on the non-LLI plot represent outliers; there are none in the LLI group. An extreme value SPSS recognizes as over 3 times the length of the box away from the box; there are none in these plots. As you can see from Figure 6.1, the LLI values are more spread out than the non-LLI values and have substantially lower medians and lower interquartile figures.

6.4 THE NORMAL DISTRIBUTION

In the last chapter and a half we have looked at ways of describing our data. However, many statistical tests we shall come on to in the second half of the book have a number of assumptions about the type of distribution the data comes from. Such tests are called parametric tests. Those that have no assumptions about the underlying distribution of the data are called non-parametric tests. In Chapter 5 we spent some time studying frequency distributions. These describe the shape of the distribution and the most common, and most important, shape is that described by the normal distribution. This distribution is also known as the Gaussian distribution after the German mathematician Carl Friedrich Gauss, who produced much of the early work on it.

6.4.1 Describing the normal distribution

The normal distribution is a bell-shaped curve in which the horizontal axis represents all possible values of a variable and the vertical axis the probability of those values occurring. The histogram in Figure 6.2 is an approximately normal distribution, although not perfect. If we drew a line through the centre of the tops of each of the bars of a histogram that is a perfectly normal distribution we would get the bell-shaped curve shown in Figure 6.3.

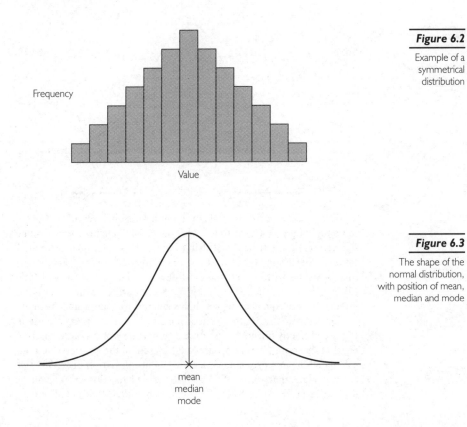

Frequency

Value

Figure 6.2

Example of a symmetrical distribution

Figure 6.3

The shape of the normal distribution, with position of mean, median and mode

mean
median
mode

The tails of the normal distribution fall off quickly and so there are few outliers. The most common values are at the centre of the distribution with the values getting rarer the further we move from this middle point. Also, the symmetry of the distribution determines that the mean, the median and the mode are at the same place, the point of symmetry, as indicated in Figure 6.3. The standard deviation is also important in the normal distribution. The point of inflexion – i.e. the point where the curve starts falling less steeply – is 1 standard deviation away from the mean. To find the point of inflexion, try tracing the bell-shaped curve in Figure 6.3 until you can feel the shift in steepness as the curve falls from the top. The mean fixes the centre of the curve, the standard deviation determines the shape of the curve. The smaller the standard deviation, the less the data spreads out from the mean; the curve will be less spread out and more peaked. There are many different normal distribution curves, based on different combinations of values for the mean and standard deviation.

A property of a perfect normal distribution is that 68% of the data will be located within 1 standard deviation of the mean, 95% within 2 standard deviations of the mean (1.96, to be more exact) and 99% within 2.58 standard deviations of the mean. In Figure 6.4 the mean is assumed to be zero and the values are measured by standard deviations away from the mean. The shaded area accounts for 95% of the data.

Figure 6.4

Normal distribution, with shaded region accounting for 95% of the data

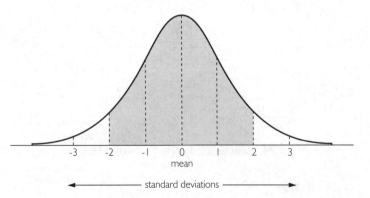

The area under the normal curve, therefore, encloses all (100%) of the data. There is a probability of 0.68 (a 68% chance) that a value selected randomly from this distribution will be within plus or minus 1 standard deviation of the mean, a probability of 0.95 (95% chance) that it will be within 1.96 standard deviations of the mean and 0.99 (99% chance) that it will be within 2.58 standard deviations. This has important consequences, as we shall see later, for significance testing.

Let us assume that the General Health scores for people with an LLI are perfectly normally distributed (it may be worth reading section 6.5.3 at this point, before progressing). Based on this property and our calculated mean score of 45.752 and standard deviation of 22.891, we can calculate that the central 95% of scores for this group will be $45.752 \pm (1.96 \times 22.891)$; i.e. in the range (0.9, 90.6). This covers virtually the whole possible range of scores – as you would expect, first of all because we are looking at all but 5% of the respondents and secondly on the basis of the boxplot in Figure 6.1. The middle 95% of respondents actually score in the range (10, 90) so the calculation based on the assumption of a 'perfect normal distribution' is not far out.

Many distributions follow the normal distribution (and these include human characteristics such as weight, height, even examination results), but many do not. The classic non-normal distribution is income. There are a small number of high earners (chairmen of companies, sports stars, entertainers, for example) who earn considerably more than everyone else and these people skew the income distribution towards the higher end of the income scale. An example of a skewed distribution is shown in Figure 6.5. This is called a positive skew as the tail is to the right, i.e. most values are at the lower end of the scale, with a few higher values pulling out the tail to the upper or right end of the distribution.

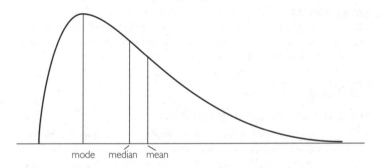

mode   median   mean

Figure 6.5

Example of skewed distribution, with approximate position of the mean, median and mode

The locations of the mean, median and mode for this skewed distribution are also shown in Figure 6.5. Remember, a skewed distribution could be skewed in the opposite direction, with most values towards the top end of the scale, a negative skew.

6.4.2 The standard normal distribution

This is a special distribution that usefully provides a standard way to present normally distributed data. It has the following characteristics:

- it is a normal distribution;
- it has a mean of 0;
- it has a standard deviation of 1.

It is also known as the Z distribution.

Observations from a normal distribution are often expressed in standard deviation units about the mean based on this Z distribution. This is called a 'standard score' and is calculated as follows:

$$\text{standard score} = \frac{\text{observed score} - \text{mean}}{\text{standard deviation}}$$

It is also known as a Z score.

We can turn any normal distribution into a Z distribution, e.g. the scores for females aged between 18 and 64 without an LLI, assuming they are normally distributed. The mean Physical Functioning scale score for this group is 72.3; standard deviation is 20.5. Miss Fit has scored 95 on this scale; we shall re-score this as a standard score: (95 − 72.3) / 20.5 = 1.11. By studying Table B1 in Appendix B and by looking down the column under 'standard score' until we get to the figure 1.11, we can see that this relates to around about the 87th percentile; hence approximately 87% of our sample of females aged 18–64 have scored below Miss Fit. She, therefore, scores near the top end of our scale.

Note that none of what we have talked about in section 6.4 (and, indeed, most of this chapter) relates to categorical data. It is nonsensical to calculate means, standard deviations and medians for nominal and most ordinal data (although, as previously stated, it is sometimes performed for some ordinal data).

6.5 THE PRACTICALITIES

6.5.1 Is your data normally distributed?

There are a number of ways to check to see if your data is approximately normally distributed or not. The first thing to do is to assess the symmetry of the data; drawing a histogram is a good idea and overlaying it with a normal curve based on the mean and standard deviation can be done by some computer packages such as SPSS for Windows. You can then assess whether the normal curve 'fits' the histogram.

Ask yourself:

• Are positive and negative deviations from the centre of the distribution equally likely?

• Do values become more unlikely (rarer) the further they tend from the centre?

The closeness of the mean to the median is another way of checking approximately for symmetry, since they should be very similar if the distribution is normal. Furthermore, in a symmetrical distribution, the lower and upper quartiles should be equidistant from the median. Bear in mind, however, that a symmetrical distribution need not be normal. A uniform distribution is symmetrical but all values are equally possible, unlike the normal distribution where values close to the mean are more likely.

Other methods will only be outlined here but further information on them can be obtained from many statistical texts, such as Altman (1991). They include the drawing of a normal probability plot (available in most statistical packages), where values are plotted against what their expected value would be if it was actually normally distributed. To be from a normal distribution the data should fit on a reasonably straight line.

A value known as the **skewness** tells us how skewed the curve is. The closer to zero the value for the skewness is, the more symmetrical is the distribution. A positive value indicates a positive skewness (i.e. a skewness to the right). A value can be calculated called the **kurtosis** and this tells us how peaked the distribution is. A positive value for kurtosis indicate that the distribution is more peaked than normal, a negative value indicates that it is less peaked (or flatter) than normal. Again, for the distribution to be normal, we would expect the value for kurtosis to be around zero. The usefulness and interpretation of these values is somewhat debatable and no more will be said about them here. For more details see Pett (1997).

Other tests detect how close a distribution is to normality. These include the Shapiro–Wilk W test and the Kolmogorov–Smirnov test. These, however, should also be used with caution (see Pett, 1997)

6.5.2 When to use different descriptive statistics

If you are reasonably confident that your data can approximate a normal distribution then the mean and standard deviation are the statistics to emphasize. An alternative to the standard deviation, although based on it, are confidence intervals for the mean, which will take our attention in Chapter 8. These statistics make more use of the data (as do tests that rely on the normal distribution) than do the median and other tests. It is also worth getting into the habit of reporting the median alongside the mean so that readers can get some idea of the symmetry of the distribution. If the data is skewed then the median and the five number summary are more appropriate. These would then lead on to non-parametric tests, i.e. those not having an underlying assumption about the distribution from which the data is taken. For categorical data, the mode, alongside other frequency and percentage values, is used.

What is of prime concern is that you look directly at the characteristics that your data possess and assess which average best represents the data for the use to which you intend to put it.

6.5.3 The normal distribution and the SF-36

Most of this chapter has used scales of the SF-36 to exemplify the normal distribution and its properties. Although the majority of work performed with the SF-36 and the papers published on it have concentrated on reporting the mean and standard deviation and using tests that assume a normal distribution, it is possible to argue that the scales are not normally distributed. Indeed, certain scales such as Role Limitations due to Physical Health (RP) and Role Limitations due to

Emotional Health (RE) appear to be non-normal. They have 'floor and ceiling effects' whereby most people tend to score at the lowest or highest end of the scale. The histograms of Physical Functioning (PF) in Figure 5.4 seem to show few of the properties of the normal distribution. You will notice that we constantly use the phrase 'assuming a normal distribution' when starting examples. A perfect normal distribution is extremely rare and our large sample size in the LLI study means we can use the central limit theorem, which will be discussed in Chapter 8. It is up to you to decide how reasonable it is to assume a normal distribution from your data and which tests are most appropriate for your needs.

6.6 FURTHER THOUGHTS ON DESCRIPTIVE ANALYSIS

It is good to develop the habit of reporting the median even if you think the mean and standard deviation are appropriate. Table 6.3 gives a clear summary of the SF-36 scales using the mean and standard deviation and the median and lower and upper quartiles.

Table 6.3

Summary of the SF-36 scale scores

		n	Mean (SD)	Lower quartile	Median	Upper quartile
General Health	LLI	569	45.8 (22.89)	30.0	45.0	62.0
	Non-LLI	584	75.0 (17.62)	65.0	77.0	87.0
Physical Functioning	LLI	587	49.3 (31.55)	20.0	50.0	80.0
	Non-LLI	584	86.8 (19.12)	85.0	95.0	100.0
Bodily Pain	LLI	583	49.1 (27.65)	31.0	41.0	72.0
	Non-LLI	589	80.9 (22.10)	72.0	84.0	100.0
Role Limitation – Physical	LLI	538	37.4 (43.25)	0.0	0.0	100.0
	Non-LLI	577	86.8 (27.54)	100.0	100.0	100.0
Role Limitation – Emotional	LLI	536	58.8 (45.60)	0.0	100.0	100.0
	Non-LLI	584	85.2 (29.91)	100.0	100.0	100.0
Social Functioning	LLI	580	64.3 (31.09)	38.9	69.4	100.0
	Non-LLI	590	91.3 (16.98)	80.0	88.9	100.0
Vitality	LLI	580	44.5 (22.05)	31.3	43.8	62.5
	Non-LLI	589	65.3 (18.43)	56.3	68.8	75.0
Mental Health	LLI	581	67.2 (20.08)	55.0	70.0	81.3
	Non-LLI	591	76.5 (16.59)	70.0	80.0	90.0

n is the number of cases where a scale score was able to be calculated.

As you can see, there appears to be a big difference between the scores for those with LLI and those without for all the scales, although the Mental Health scale is closest to being equal between the LLI and non-LLI groups. Furthermore, the means and medians are reasonably similar, except for the two Role Limitations scales, which are the ones with the floor and ceiling effects.

The next step now is to move to thinking about whether having an LLI is the only reason for the difference in scores or whether there are other factors that may explain the difference. Such alternative explanations are called **confounders**. An example is that the LLI group has a larger proportion of the older age groups among its number (mean 62.4, SD 14.20 compared to mean 54.6, SD 15.18 for the non-LLI group). Age is therefore a possible confounding factor that needs to be taken into consideration in the main analysis. Common knowledge tells us that the older age groups are likely to have worse health and, therefore, to score worse on the SF-36 (as has been shown by, for example, Brazier et al. (1992), except for the Mental Health scale). Gender is another potential confounder.

Another step is to notice the wider spread of scores in the group with an LLI. In other words, they have a higher standard deviation. While the non-LLI group should contain reasonably healthy people (apart from those with short-term illnesses), the LLI group will contain people with a wide range of conditions, which is likely to be reflected by differences in their health profile scores.

There are more 'sophisticated' ways of exploring the effect of confounding variables than the one we are about to show but it is an easy way of exploring differences in subgroups. In Table 6.4 we have simply divided the population into conventional sex- age groups to compare results.

We have taken the scale GH as an example. As you can see, as age increases the SF-36 scores do decrease but it appears that there is still

		n	Mean (SD)	Lower quartile	Median	Upper quartile
Total	LLI	569	45.8 (22.89)	30.0	45.0	62.0
	Non-LLI	584	75.0 (17.62)	65.0	77.0	87.0
F18–44	LLI	33	53.9 (22.91)	36.0	50.0	77.0
	Non-LLI	60	78.0 (17.55)	72.0	82.0	92.0
F45–64	LLI	127	45.4 (21.92)	30.0	42.0	65.0
	Non-LLI	168	76.4 (17.00)	67.0	80.0	87.0
F65–74	LLI	86	49.6 (19.21)	35.0	47.0	62.0
	Non-LLI	52	73.0 (15.27)	62.0	72.0	87.0
F75+	LLI	68	37.1 (20.83)	20.0	32.5	50.0
	Non-LLI	31	73.3 (17.53)	62.0	77.0	87.0
M18–44	LLI	29	57.0 (26.97)	35.0	62.0	81.0
	Non-LLI	54	78.2 (18.42)	66.5	82.0	91.0
M45–64	LLI	117	43.6 (24.16)	25.0	40.0	67.0
	Non-LLI	146	74.5 (18.42)	65.0	77.0	90.0
M65–74	LLI	82	47.6 (23.89)	25.0	47.5	67.0
	Non-LLI	56	69.2 (19.25)	57.0	72.0	82.0
M75+	LLI	27	38.4 (29.58)	25.0	40.0	52.0
	Non-LLI	17	71.5 (11.20)	62.0	72.0	79.5

Table 6.4

Summary of the General Health scale score by age and sex

n is the number of cases where a scale score was able to be calculated.

a difference between LLI and non-LLI groups. Gender does not seem to have such a big effect as age. Stratifying the data and inspecting the results in this way is a simple first step in exploring confounding factors.

6.7 DESCRIPTIVE OUTPUT FROM SPSS FOR WINDOWS

Using a summary statistics command in a statistical package can often mean producing a jumble of tables to help a decision over which of the statistics are actually needed. In this section we shall look at the output commonly given from statistical packages using SPSS for Windows as our example. The output is from SPSS for Windows for the General Health (GH) scale from the SF-36 from our LLI survey. There are actually three ways of obtaining summary statistics using SPSS for Windows; the FREQUENCIES command, the DESCRIPTIVES command and the EXPLORE command. The DESCRIPTIVES command gives us much the same information as the other two except for the fact that it does not give the percentiles or the median and mode, which is why we tend to use either the FREQUENCIES command or the EXPLORE command. The EXPLORE command can either be used with the whole data (as we have so far done with GH), or the data can be split up into groups.

An analysis in which we looked at the General Health scores in total would be misleading as it covers two different groups: the LLI group and the non-LLI group. It would be more informative to look at the descriptive data of the two groups separately; as we did with the histograms in Figure 5.5.

Table 6.5 shows output from the EXPLORE command, using just the 'Descriptives' subcommand, broken down by the presence or absence of LLI.

We shall consider the data for the non-LLI group and leave it to you to study the LLI group and consider the differences.

'Valid cases' tells us for how many cases (or for how many respondents) a scale score could be calculated for the GH scale. On the SF-36, remember, there are a number of questions on each scale and scores from these questions can be summed and transformed into one scale score for each question. Scale scores were calculated if over half the questions on that scale were answered, so for 584 respondents in the non-LLI group scores could be calculated and for 18 people they could not ('Missing cases'). This gives us our total response of 602 respondents and the percentage of missing cases is $(18 / 602) \times 100 = 3.0\%$ ('Percent missing'). Normally 'Valid cases' are those for which answers, or 'values', were obtained; e.g. all the times a particular question was answered on a questionnaire

The 'Mean' is given as 74.9693. This, as we know from earlier, is the sum of values divided by the number of 'Valid cases'. The mean is close to the 'Median' (77.000), which indicates that the distribution is reasonably symmetrical. As you can see, both statistics are much higher than those for the LLI group. We do not need hypothesis tests to tell

GH   general health
By   LLI   0   no

Table 6.5

Descriptive data for
the General Health
(GH) SF-36 scale by
reporting of a LLI or
not

Valid cases: 584.0   Missing cases: 18.0   Percent missing: 3.0

Mean	74.9693	Std Err	0.7291	Min	0.0000	Skewness	−0.5002
Median	77.0000	Variance	310.4666	Max	100.0000	S E Skew	0.1011
5% Trim	76.0119	Std Dev	17.6201	Range	100.0000	Kurtosis	0.6709
95% CI for Mean	(73.5373, 76.4013)			IQR	22.0000	SE Kurt	0.2019

Percentiles

Percentiles	5.0000	10.0000	25.0000	50.0000	75.0000	90.0000	95.0000
Score	41.2500	52.0000	65.0000	77.0000	87.0000	97.0000	100.0000

GH   general health
By   LLI   1   yes

Valid cases: 569.0   Missing cases: 34.0   Percent missing: 5.6

Mean	45.7516	Std Err	0.9596	Min	0.0000	Skewness	0.1825
Median	45.0000	Variance	524.0068	Max	100.0000	S E Skew	0.1024
5% Trim	45.5151	Std Dev	22.8912	Range	100.0000	Kurtosis	−0.6992
95% CI for Mean	(43.8667, 47.6365)			IQR	32.0000	SE Kurt	0.2045

Percentiles

Percentiles	5.0000	10.0000	25.0000	50.0000	75.0000	90.0000	95.0000
Score	10.0000	15.0000	30.0000	45.0000	62.0000	77.0000	82.8750

us that there is a difference in the mean scores between those reporting an LLI and those who reported no LLI as the difference is so large (74.9693 compared to 45.7516) – another example of the usefulness of descriptive analyses.

Other figures we can recognize include 'Variance', which is 310.467. If we take the square root of this, i.e. √310.467, we get 17.620 (the 'Std Dev' or standard deviation). Notice that the LLI group has a greater variability of scores than the non-LLI as pointed out earlier. We can see from the scores for the minimum ('Min' – 0) and the maximum ('Max' – 100) that the scores cover the full range from 0–100 (remember, the possible scores range from 0–100 on the SF-36 for each scale). The 'Range' is also given; it is 100, i.e. from 0–100. If the range stretched below zero or above 100 (i.e. if the minimum score had been less than zero or the maximum had been greater than 100) we would have realized that a mistake had been made somewhere and that would 'instruct' us to go back and check the data. Ask yourself whether the data makes sense. Of course, the range need not have stretched as far as 0 or 100.

If you look down to the 'Percentiles' underneath, you will recognize the 50th percentile as the median (hence, it has the same value as the median of 77.000) and the 25th and 75th as the lower and upper quartile respectively. These values are 65.000 for the lower quartile and 87.000 for the upper quartile. This means that 25% of the scores fell at or below 65 and 75% at or below 87. If we take the lower quartile figure from the upper quartile figure, we get 22.000. This is the interquartile range ('IQR'). The upper and lower quartiles are reasonably similar distances from the median, which again suggests a symmetrical distribution. There is a range of scores but they get less frequent as we move from the mean, as in Figure 5.5b.

Go back to the boxplot in Figure 6.1 and you will see how the plot has been constructed using these figures.

The middle 80% of people score between 52 and 97 (between the 10th and 90th percentiles).

There are a number of other figures. 'Std Err', or the standard error of the mean, will be taken up in Chapter 8. The four figures on the right-hand side tell us more about the frequency curve of the data and have already been mentioned briefly. The 'Skewness' and its standard error ('S E Skew') tell us how skewed the curve is. The 'Kurtosis' and its standard error ('S E Kurt') tell us how peaked the distribution is.

The value '5% Trim' is another way of calculating the mean mentioned previously. This is the trimmed mean and is used when outliers (or extreme observations) are suspected. The 5% tells us that the smallest 5% and the largest 5% have been removed and the mean has been calculated from the remaining 90% of values. This is sometimes preferred to the median when extreme values are suspected because it makes more use of the data than the median but, like the median, should be less affected by outlying observations. In this case, the trimmed means are not so dissimilar to the means and so we can work on the mean and assume there are very few or no outliers.

The figure labelled '95% CI for Mean' is the 95% confidence interval for the mean, something we shall concentrate more on in Chapter 8.

6.8 NUMBER OF SIGNIFICANT DIGITS

One thing you may have noticed from Table 6.5 is that the EXPLORE command gives results to four decimal places. By contrast, the FRE-QUENCIES command, if we were to use it, gives output to three decimal places. It is down to you when you report the results to decide to how many significant digits to take your results. You do not want to put people off by quoting an excessive number of digits, but neither do you want to detract from the accuracy of your data. Bear in mind that the phrase 'significant digits' refers to something different from what is meant by 'decimal places'. Significant digits (or figures) are the number of digits relevant to the number's precision. For example, we obtained answers from 2867 people in the first stage of our survey. We could have rounded this to 2870 people (three significant digits) or 2900 (two significant digits) or 3000 (one significant digit). Each reduction in the number of significant digits reduces the accuracy.

Altman *et al.* (1983) suggest that percentages be quoted normally to only one decimal place and means to only one decimal place more than the measurements of the raw data itself. Standard deviations and standard errors can be extended to one extra decimal place. So, in our study, age has always been stated to two significant figures and no decimal places (in effect, rounded to the nearest whole figure) so we would quote the mean to one decimal place and standard deviation to two. For the GH scores above, both the mean and standard deviation could be quoted reasonably to two decimal places.

When data needs to be extremely accurate, perhaps when further calculations are to be performed on it and where rounding off could give misleading results, more digits might be needed.

The method of rounding off is simple. Digits not required are dropped if the first one in line is less than 5. If the first digit to be dropped is 5 or higher, then the last remaining digit is increased by 1. So, the mean for the non-LLI group for the GH scale score is 74.9693 from Table 6.5. Rounding to three decimal places gives 74.969, two decimal places gives 74.97 and one decimal place is 75.0. Try reducing the mean for the LLI group (45.7516) to three, two and one decimal places and then both means to one significant place. The answers are at the end of this chapter. Remember, figures should only be rounded for reporting, not during analysis.

6.9 CHECKING DATA QUALITY – REVISITED

The summaries given in Table 6.5 are another method for the suspiciously or pessimistically minded to check for any obvious mistakes in the data. We know that all the scale scores for the SF-36 range from 0–100 so the minimum and maximum must be between 0 and 100; if not there has been a mistake somewhere along the way.

Similarly, if the mean was outside the range 0–100 we would know there had been some kind of error in the data. Once again, common sense is very important. It is not just a matter of telling the computer to do an analysis and recording it, but also of interpreting the results and applying common sense to the interpretation of them.

6.10 SUMMARY

In this chapter we have started the process of analysing interval and ratio data using averages and measures of variability. We have also introduced the important concept of the normal distribution, which will be a common theme for the rest of this book. A basic report or paper will contain some form of descriptive analysis even if it does not move on to the inferential statistics of the next chapters, and this will be either in the form of percentages and graphs or of averages and measures of variability.

The last two chapters have concentrated on helping you to understand your data and prepare it for future investigations, and, as such, they were preparations for the way ahead, both in this book and in data analysis.

6.11 ANSWERS TO EXERCISE

The figure 45.7516 rounded to three decimal places is 45.752, to two decimal places 45.75 and to one decimal place 45.8. To one significant figure it would be 50 and 74.9693 to one significant figure is 70. Note the amount of lost information the fewer decimal places or significant figures we use.

7 SIGNPOSTS AND CROSSROADS FOR THE REST OF THE BOOK

7.1 INTRODUCTION

In this chapter we wish to take stock of where things have got to so far and what is to come in the next part of the book. In particular we wish to highlight a few key areas that we think are important for those not trained in statistics to grasp and understand in order to make the choice of how to approach the analysis of their data. In the second part of the book there are a number of more detailed, technically more difficult parts, which you may decide to read or not dependent upon your data or your willingness to get involved in statistical analysis. The important issue is to understand where each section fits in to the whole picture, and what the basis is for choosing to go down one particular road or not.

7.2 SUMMARIZING YOUR DATA

The function of the previous two chapters of the book has been to introduce you to the first, most important but often (for the non-statistician) least appreciated part of statistics – the rules for summarizing data.

You have learned about different types of data and different distributions of data and how this leads to choices of summary of the centre of your data – means or medians, for example – and of the pattern and extremes of your data – standard deviations or ranges, for example.

A key idea to grasp here is that, when you enter the statistical, mathematical world, you are moving into an artificial world of rules and laws. These help us to hold a mirror up to the real world and within that reflected image to move forward logically and make deductions by following the rules of the game. The 'normal distribution' is a mathematical construction whose world we enter because it follows rules that help us to manage, summarize and deduce things in a standard way that can be communicated to others. Height, for example, tends to approximate to the normal distribution and play by its rules. Even if our actual data is not normally distributed, we may be able to invoke the central limit theorem (to be explained in Chapter 8), if this is valid for our situation, to enter the normal distribution world. Or we may abandon the attempt and choose another set of rules in which to move with our data (the non-parametric situation, for example).

7.3 IMPORTANT IDEAS 1 – SAMPLES AND POPULATIONS

If the purpose of our data gathering were to do no more than summarize our own particular group of subjects – the patients we saw this morning or the clients who phoned in during the last month – we would stop there. So we might have the average age of the patients, or the number who are female, or those who have a limiting long-term illness (LLI). If this were simply an exercise in, say, planning a service for this group and for no-one else, this might be fine. 'I want to post everyone who phoned me last month a booklet about services in our practice'. All you want to know is the total count of those who phoned and target these with the special version of the booklet for those with chronic illness.

Research, however, almost always takes you further than this. You are usually gathering data to make inferences about some wider group of subjects (or **population**) to which the results from your sample might apply, or to make comparisons with other populations elsewhere. 'Population' here is not used in the everyday sense of a nation or town, it is literally any group of people or **units** of which your own study sample is made up (it could be animals, events, things, for example).

Just think for a moment what you are doing if you convert the number of people with LLI who have been to see you in the last month into a percentage. You do not need to do this for your task of sending out booklets, because for that you simply need to know the actual number. It feels natural, though, in 'summarizing' or writing or talking about it to state that '20% of my patients last month had LLI'. Why? Because very often providing a service is a continuing thing – how many booklets 'on average' might you need to supply in the next few months, for example? Or, you might wish to give other practitioners an estimate of the proportion of LLI patients they might have in their practice. Or, you might want to compare with the practice up the road and ask 'Are they different?'

The logical pitfalls of doing this have already been discussed in the survey chapter, Chapter 3. For example, was the last month typical? Did I ascertain everyone with an LLI or might I have missed some? Is my practice likely to be different from others with respect to the frequency of LLI; for example, is my practice population older (it might, for instance, be situated in a seaside retirement town)?

Apart from this **logic** of comparison and extrapolation from your data, the statistical issues are also about the fact that your data is now taken to be a sample of all possible data of a similar sort. It may be taken as a sample of all patients in your practice (a **finite** population; you can define it and you know how large it is) or it may be taken, when comparing it to other practices, as a sample of a much larger population. All these other comparator populations are similarly seen as samples of a larger population (all practice populations in the UK, for example).

Many statistical ideas arise from the notion that the data we collect in a study is obtained from a sample of a much larger population.

If, for example, we wished to estimate the prevalence of LLI for the whole of the UK from a small random sample of the UK population, we have to envisage that our sample is one of many possible samples that might have been taken, as shown in Figure 7.1.

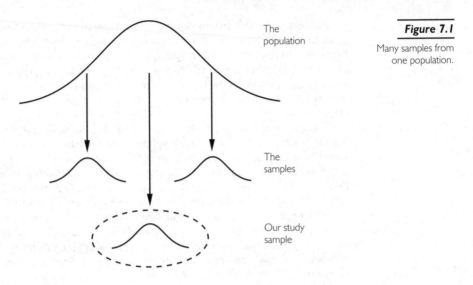

Figure 7.1

Many samples from
one population.

The
population

The
samples

Our study
sample

If each of those samples is truly 'random' (e.g. they are not drawn
from different age-groups or different social classes), then the results
obtained from the samples will vary in a way that can be predicted by
statistical 'laws'. In practice we do not take lots of samples, but we
apply the 'laws' to our one study sample.

- If our sample is a biased representation of the population we are
  hoping to characterize, there is nothing statistics can do about it.
  For example, LLI prevalence measured in a sample of over-70-
  year-olds in a working class suburb cannot represent LLI
  prevalence in all adults in the UK.

- Which population the sample represents depends on the purpose
  of the study and the sample chosen.

- The summary statistics (e.g. mean and standard deviation) of our
  sample can be taken to represent the summary statistics (both
  average and variation) of the population. The extent of the error
  in that assumption (the extent to which, assuming no bias, our
  sample summary may deviate from the population summary
  because of random variation) is called the **sampling error**. It is
  determined by sample size and the variation in the study
  measurements.

7.4 INFERENCE, ESTIMATION AND HYPOTHESIS TESTING

This notion of a much wider population of which your sample is a
small part is a crucial notion in statistics. In the survey chapter we were
often asking the question 'Is my sample representative of the population I am studying?' Given that the logic of representativeness has been
sorted out (e.g. are survey non-responders likely to be different from
responders?), we would like to estimate how confident we are that our

sample means or proportions represent the population to which we want to extrapolate our result. Chapter 8 starts to explore ways in which we can put figures to this. This approach states 'Here is our sample estimate; this is the best estimate we have of the mean or proportion in the population; how far might our sample estimate be from the true population mean or proportion?' We estimate the influence of sampling variation.

Much of medical and health services research consists of comparing two or more samples (perhaps subpopulations from one sample survey) and asking 'Are they different?' What we are actually doing (after thinking about the logic of the comparison – are we comparing like with like? Is there any bias?), is asking how confident can we be that these two samples come from the same population (i.e. any differences that have arisen are due to sampling variation) or that they come from different populations (i.e. any differences are real). Once again we can approach this as an estimation by summarizing the difference between the sample groups and estimating the likely influence of sampling error on this difference.

There is a whole range of statistical approaches that take this a step further. These are called **hypothesis tests**. The hypothesis test starts from the point of view that both study samples are from the same population, 'the hypothesis of no difference', e.g. that the samples have identical means. The tests then provide an estimate of the probability that the hypothesis is false – the probability that the samples come from different populations and that differences between them have not arisen because of sampling variation. The second part of Chapter 8 and Chapters 9 and 10 guide you through the welter of hypothesis tests. How to choose which test to use?

Well, reading through the chapters gives the necessary basis for doing this, but the detail can be a bit alarming at times for the non-statistician, and so we have summarized some signposts for you, displayed in Figure 7.2 with the relevant sections of the book.

Remember, that parametric tests (those based on the assumption of the normal distribution or where use of the central limit theorem is viable) still have some other assumptions, which will be stated in the relevant sections later in the book. If these assumptions cannot be met, we may need to use non-parametric tests, although we prefer to use the parametric equivalents (see section 9.2 for reasons why). The parametric test for each situation, as well as its non-parametric equivalent, is given.

Remember, however, that the logic comes first. If you have a sample of 18–30-year-olds, they cannot represent 50-year-olds. If you have a sample in which 50% have not sent back your questionnaire, you need some estimate of whether the 50% non-responders might have different characteristics relevant to the topic of the questionnaire before you start considering issues of sampling variation.

But after the logic, the statistics of estimation and hypothesis testing can be brought into play. There are clear signposts to finding your way through, revealed in Figure 7.2.

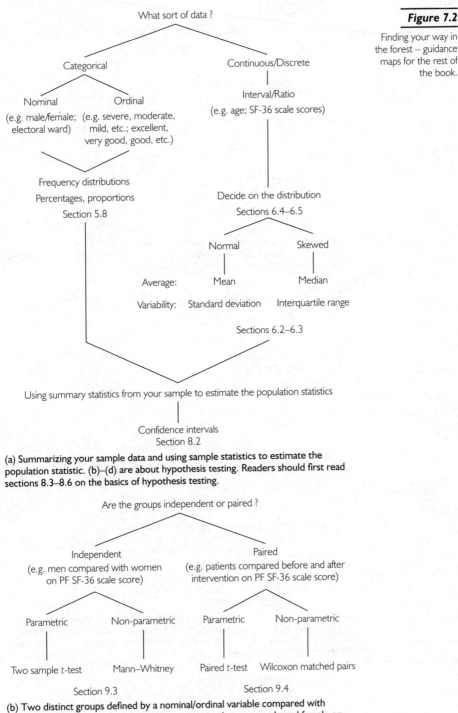

Figure 7.2

Finding your way in the forest – guidance maps for the rest of the book.

(a) Summarizing your sample data and using sample statistics to estimate the population statistic. (b)–(d) are about hypothesis testing. Readers should first read sections 8.3–8.6 on the basics of hypothesis testing.

(b) Two distinct groups defined by a nominal/ordinal variable compared with respect to an interval/ratio variable (e.g. comparing between male and female on Physical Functioning SF-36 scale score).

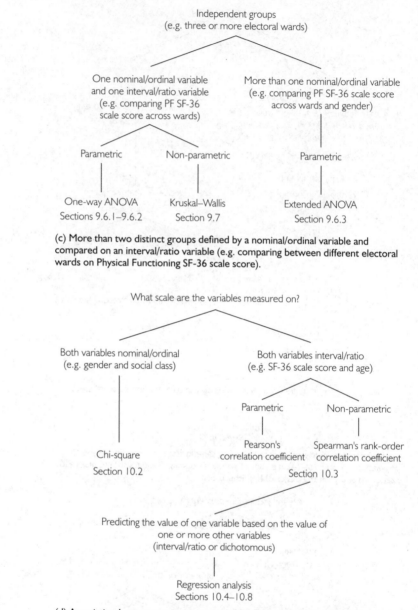

(c) **More than two distinct groups defined by a nominal/ordinal variable and compared on an interval/ratio variable** (e.g. comparing between different electoral wards on Physical Functioning SF-36 scale score).

(d) **Association between two or more variables from sample measured on same measurement scale** (e.g. comparing gender with social class; Physical Functioning SF-36 scale score and age); predicting the value of one variable based on the value of one or more other variables.

8 STARTING TO DRAW INFERENCES FROM YOUR DATA

8.1 INTRODUCTION

We are now going to enter the arena of **inferential** statistics. Here the procedure of drawing conclusions about our study population begins, based on the sample data. What can we actually determine about the population?

In this chapter we look at a way of showing how accurate we believe our data is, and how much confidence we can put in this accuracy. We also start looking at hypothesis testing, what it is and what it is not, and what exactly does that 'p-value' mean, on which so much seems to hang and which pops up regularly in journal articles? This will set us up for the next chapter, which will to start consider different statistical tests.

It is all-important to concentrate on our starting hypothesis, on the purpose of the survey, and not to get side-tracked. It is easy to go down alleyways to explore what look like 'interesting' questions. However, what we can infer depends heavily on why we started the project in the first place.

In Chapters 5 and 6 we have tried to characterize what was typical in our sample survey respondents and how these individuals differed in terms of the characteristics under investigation. Now, in this chapter and in the following two chapters, we shall expand this to look at what is typical in the study population, how widely individuals in the population differ, and to try and extrapolate our data from our sample to the population. We shall consider how to detect differences between subgroups of the population and how to assess whether the sample data support our expectations and starting hypotheses or not. We will consider how to select the appropriate statistical test and how to interpret the results. In a later chapter, relationships between variables will be tackled also, for example, how weight varies with height in human beings.

8.1.1 Important ideas 2 – the central limit theorem

The assumption that our sample data comes from an approximately normal distribution is crucial to many statistical techniques. An important – and remarkable – theorem helps us here. It is worthwhile (but a little tricky) trying to grasp what this important theorem (called the central limit theorem) is all about.

Suppose there were lots of different studies of LLI going on around the country and each of them was attempting to estimate the prevalence of LLI for the country's population as a whole. Let us assume that each of the studies takes a random sample of the population. There will then be a whole series of different random samples of the population of the country, each with an estimate of the population LLI. We could then plot these sample estimates of the population prevalence and obtain the distribution of these sample estimates of LLI. This is called the 'sampling distribution'.

Figure 8.1

The idea of the
central limit theorem

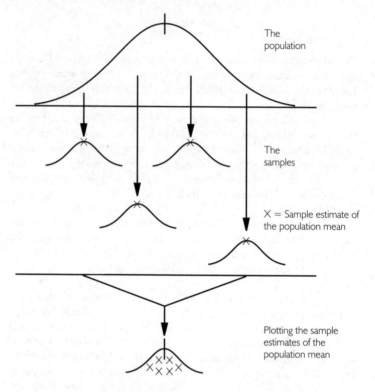

The
population

The
samples

X = Sample estimate of
the population mean

Plotting the sample
estimates of the
population mean

The central limit theorem reveals a number of things about this sampling distribution that are very intriguing and very helpful to statistics.

- If we draw a histogram of all the sample estimates, it would fall into the shape of a normal distribution.

- The larger the size of the samples, the closer the sampling distribution will be to a normal distribution.

This works for different sample statistics, such as the mean. If we drew repeated samples from the same population and calculated the mean each time, the histogram of those means would form a normal distribution as in Figure 8.1.

This signifies that, for large sample sizes, we are able to use the central limit theorem as validation for using parametric tests (i.e. reliant on normal distribution assumptions). This applies even to sample data that is non-normal from small samples. For symmetrical data, the sample size only needs to be greater than 30 or 40 for this to happen; for very skewed distributions, the sample size will need to be comfortably over 100.

It works with proportions too, such as the LLI prevalence. Our sample estimate of LLI prevalence is based on each person ('sampling unit') having or not having the characteristic (LLI) – this is a binomial distribution as there are two possible outcomes. If our sample is seen as one of many possible samples that estimate population prevalence for our study population, the distribution of those estimates would fall into a normal distribution.

It is important to realize that the sampling distribution is a theoretical distribution: 'What would happen if we took lots of samples from the same population and calculated the same statistic each time and then plotted the distribution of all those sample statistics?' We do not actually do this – but we can base a number of calculations and ideas on it. Most importantly, it leads us to the calculation of the standard error of our sample estimate (for example, the mean).

In our theoretical world of sample means forming a normal distribution, that distribution will have a 'standard deviation'– the variation in those means. This 'standard deviation' of all the sample means is called the **standard error of the mean** , and is our measure of the error involved in studying a single sample rather than a whole population.

A single sample of a particular size and with a particular spread of data will generate, as we will see, a particular measure of this standard or sampling error.

8.2 HOW CONFIDENT CAN WE BE IN OUR ESTIMATES?

8.2.1 What is a confidence interval?

In Chapter 6 we presented a mean for the General Health (GH) scale of the Short Form-36 (SF-36) for the limiting long-term illness (LLI) group. This mean can be considered a **point estimate** of the mean GH scale score for all those who would report an LLI registered with the general practice concerned, i.e. an estimate of the mean for the population as a whole. However, we cannot say with total confidence that this point estimate is exactly the same as the actual mean for our study population. As we have only taken a sample rather than studied the whole population, it would be unlikely that we have estimated the population mean exactly because of the error involved in questioning only a sample of our population. Can we, therefore, produce a statement about how accurately our sample estimate matches the population figure?

An **interval** can be calculated, within which we would expect the population mean to lie. This gives us our degree of accuracy. Further, as we can never be 100% confident of anything, we need to put a confidence level on to this interval. We shall start by considering a confidence interval for the population mean. This estimate takes into account our sample mean and the standard deviation of the data we have collected in the sample. It assumes that the data is normally distributed or that we have a large sample size (i.e. using the central limit theorem).

If you remember, when looking at the example output from SPSS for Windows in Table 6.5 we came across a result labelled '95% CI for Mean'. This is the 95% confidence interval calculated for the mean.

8.2.2 Calculating a confidence interval for the mean

Firstly, we must assume that we will be estimating the population variance from the sample variance.

There are two ways of calculating a confidence interval: one for when the sample size is large, greater than 30, say, and one when it is small. If the sample size is large, then even if the data does not appear normally distributed the assumption of a normal distribution does not carry serious consequences.

Most computer packages will, as we saw SPSS for Windows do, give a confidence interval for the mean. But, again, you need to understand the calculation to understand more of its interpretation and its reliance on the variability of the data set as summarized by the standard deviation.

The first step is to calculate the sample mean and standard deviation. The second step is to calculate the standard error of the mean, which is simply the standard deviation divided by the square root of the sample size.

Let us start by looking at the case of a large sample size. The most frequently used levels of confidence are the 90%, 95% (the most common) and 99%. We multiply the standard error by the required figure obtained from the normal distribution table, Table B2 in Appendix B (you will start recognizing the numbers here). For the 95% level (where $\alpha = 0.05$; that is 100% − 95%) we use 1.96, for 90% (where $\alpha = 0.10$) it is 1.645 and for the 99% level (where $\alpha = 0.01$) it is 2.576. The last step is simply to add to, and subtract from, the mean to get the confidence limits.

So, for a 95% confidence interval for the population mean, μ, the formula is written as:

$$\bar{x} \pm 1.96s / \sqrt{n}.$$

You will remember that $\bar{x}$ is the sample mean, s is the sample standard deviation (our approximation to the population standard deviation) and n is the sample size. Obviously, to get a 90% or 99% confidence interval, or whatever size is required, you replace 1.96 with the relevant figure.

Let us see, then, how the confidence interval was calculated for General Health and those without limiting long-term illness in Table 6.5. The standard error is the standard deviation divided by the square root of the sample size. So, from Table 6.5, we know that the standard deviation is 17.6201 and the sample size is 584. The standard error, therefore, is 17.6201 / $\sqrt{584}$, which equals 0.7291 (which is what is stated in the table). To get a 95% confidence interval for the mean, we multiply this figure by 1.96, which gives us 1.4291. Next, we add this to our mean to get the high limit of the interval, i.e. 74.9693 + 1.4291

= 76.40 to two decimal places, and subtract from the mean to get the lower limit of the interval, i.e. 74.9693 − 1.4291 = 73.54. The interval is then written as (73.54, 76.40).

The large sample size has given us a reasonably narrow interval around the sample mean. Let us now look at a smaller sample, and now we need to believe that our data is normally distributed. Consider a study on 16 males of age 65 and over, in which their General Health mean is to be calculated, assuming that the figures come from a normal distribution. The mean turns out again to be 74.9693 and the standard deviation is again 17.6201. The standard error is 17.6201 / √16 = 4.4050. The only change to the formula described in the paragraph above is that, as the sample size is small, we need to look in a *t*-distribution table as shown in Table B3 in Appendix B. The format here is that you subtract 1 from the sample size to get a figure that is called **the degrees of freedom.** So 16 minus 1 gives 15 degrees of freedom. Then, by looking in Table B3 under 15 degrees of freedom (DF) and α = 0.05, we can see the figure given is 2.131. So, our 95% confidence interval is 74.9693 ± (2.131 × 4.4050). Hence to the limits (65.58, 84.36). Our sample size is smaller, and so the confidence interval is much wider. See for yourself what would happen if we had decided on a 90% or a 99% confidence interval (the answers are at the end of the chapter). With less confidence the interval becomes smaller; with more confidence it increases, as we want greater confidence in the population mean being included in our confidence interval. We shall return to the use and the concept of the *t*-distribution in the next chapter.

8.2.3 What does it mean?

A 95% confidence interval can be interpreted as follows. If we took a large number of random samples all of the same size from the same population and calculated a 95% confidence interval each time, then 95% of these intervals would contain the population mean. This 95% level is the most commonly used but we could have a 90% confidence level (in which case, 90% of the intervals would contain the population mean) or, perhaps, a 99% confidence level (in which case 99% of the intervals would contain the population mean). The larger the confidence level (i.e. the closer to 100% it is), the wider the interval will be since we want to be more confident about our interval enclosing the true population mean. Similarly, a smaller sample size will give a wider interval than a larger sample size, and so we need a reasonably large sample to obtain reasonably accurate results. Further, the more variability there is in the population, the wider the interval will be.

While it is not theoretically correct, the 95% confidence interval is often interpreted and understood more easily as there being a 95% probability that the population figure lies within the interval. This is not theoretically correct because the true figure will either be, or not be, within this interval so it does not make too much sense to give a probability for it. Moore (1991) suggests that one way of looking at a 95% confidence interval is that the interval was obtained by a method which gives us the correct results 95% of the time. We are 95% confident that our estimate lies within this interval.

8.2.4 Calculating a confidence interval for a proportion

It is also possible to derive confidence intervals for proportions because of the central limit theorem explained earlier. We need a large sample and a figure of 30 or more is the rather arbitrary size given in many texts. Altman (1991) suggests that the central limit theorem comes into play when p and $1 - p$ are both greater than $5 / n$ where p is the proportion and n is the sample size.

Consider the case taken from our hospital satisfaction survey. A total of 42 out of the 50 respondents rated the care they received as either excellent or very good. Let us calculate a 90% confidence interval for the proportion rating the care received as either excellent or very good; $p = 42 / 50 = 0.84$. Using Altman's rule above, we have 5 $/ n = 5 / 50 = 0.1$, which is smaller than both p and $1 - p$ so we can apply the central limit theorem. The figure needed for 90% confidence can be read from the normal distribution table, Table B2 in Appendix B, and is 1.645. The equation used for calculating confidence intervals for proportions at the 90% level is:

$$p \pm 1.645 \ \sqrt{\frac{p\,(1 - p)}{n}}$$

where n is, again, the sample size. Sometimes $(1 - p)$ is written as q. Remember the proportions must add up to 1, hence $1 - p$. We can, again, change 1.645 if we require different percentage limits.

So, our confidence interval is

$$0.84 \pm 1.645 \ \sqrt{\frac{0.84 \times 0.16}{50}} = 0.84 \pm 0.085 = (0.76, 0.93)$$

This means that, if we repeated the survey 100 times on the same population and calculated a 95% confidence interval each time, 95 of the confidence intervals would include the population proportion rating their care as Excellent or Very good. Basically, we can be pretty confident the true figure for p lies between 76% and 93%.

8.2.5 Other confidence intervals

Confidence intervals for means and proportions are not the only confidence intervals you may come across, or want to calculate. Statistical packages will often give confidence intervals for other figures. It is possible to calculate a confidence interval for the difference between two means. This gives us an interval estimate for the population difference between the means based on the difference observed in our sample data.

You may also find confidence intervals given for the population variance and for estimates of coefficients in a regression model, for example, as well as other statistics calculated on sample data. The interpretations are the same as before. For more on calculating confidence intervals for different statistics, see Gardner and Altman (1989).

8.3 HYPOTHESIS TESTING

8.3.1 Important ideas 3 – what has hypothesis testing to do with sampling error?

We have seen how we can imagine our sample as being one of many possible samples from our population, and this allows us to calculate standard errors for our estimates of the mean, for example, and hence a confidence interval for our estimate. All that hypothesis testing is doing is to reformulate that idea as a 'test' of a single population.

For example, given that we have from the Census the best estimate of LLI prevalence for the whole of the UK population, how probable is it that the prevalence of LLI in our single practice in North Staffordshire is actually different from that population figure, or that any differences between the two figures (sample and Census) have arisen from the chance variation of taking only a small sample of the whole UK population?

In other words, we have a single question to test – is LLI in our practice different from the UK as a whole? We fashion this in a particular way (the **null hypothesis**), which states that our expectation is that there is no systematic difference and that any deviation in our sample prevalence from the UK prevalence as a whole has arisen from sampling error. So we are still interested in the same thing as our confidence interval (how much sampling error?), but we are addressing a particular issue (is the sampling error enough to explain the difference?). It is very important to remember that, even if you end up with the conclusion that sampling error is unlikely to explain a difference, this does not mean there definitely is a difference – that depends on what your question relates to, bias in the way your sample was selected, and so on – all the 'non-statistical' considerations around study design and drawing logical conclusions from data.

Hypothesis testing really comes into its own when you are comparing two samples.

In a comparison of LLI in two different practices, for example, the question being asked is: 'What is the likelihood or probability that the difference we observe between the groups has arisen by chance – i.e. as a result of sampling error – rather than because there is a real difference between the groups?' In other words, are they samples from the same underlying 'population', or do they represent different 'populations'? Formulating it as a null hypothesis, it becomes 'The two practices have the same LLI prevalence because they are samples from the same population, and any difference is due to sampling error'. This is where the statistical tests come in, the choice of test depending on the question being asked and the nature and distribution of the data, but

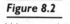

Figure 8.2

Using a sample to
infer about the
population

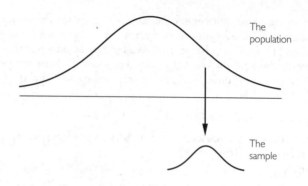

The
population

The
sample

all basically dependent on the notion of sampling error and on the central limit theorem if the sample size is large.

Remember, back at the beginning of the book we talked about the aims of projects and about hypotheses. Well, in this section we shall start along the road of testing hypotheses and assessing what it is all about: the key concepts and how to understand the notations used in articles and books, including the *p*-value. We need to perform hypothesis testing as we need to make inferences about the population from the sample.

The rest of this chapter will start to introduce the features involved in hypothesis testing, with examples using various forms of test following in Chapter 9. The remaining parts of this chapter are essential reading before Chapter 9.

8.3.2 The null and alternative hypotheses

In hypothesis testing, we normally compare our data against a standard or against a prior expectation. So, for example, we may hypothesize that the prevalence of limiting long-term illness in our study will be 24% because that is the figure obtained from Census results for North Staffordshire. Or we may expect that those with an LLI will score worse on the SF-36 than those without because logic would lead us to this conclusion provided we believe that the SF-36 is a valid measure of health status. This second hypothesis leads us on to testing between groups, which could be testing people with LLI against those without, testing between two or more drugs or testing between surgical procedures, for example. Perhaps we might hypothesize that a new drug can save more lives than the traditional drug or one treatment for cancer is better than another. Hypotheses need to be as detailed as the study demands: how should one treatment differ from another, for example? In reducing the death rate, improving symptoms, avoiding side-effects? We need to be precise as to what our endpoints are before the study begins.

The null hypothesis is a hypothesized statement usually in the form of 'No effect', or 'No difference'. The alternative hypothesis is a more general statement about an effect of a difference that we have some reason to believe might be true. The null hypothesis is usually written as H_0, and the alternative hypothesis as either H_1 or H_A. So, the following are examples of possible hypotheses:

(a) H_0: the prevalence of LLI in the population is 24% (written as $p = 0.24$ where p is the proportion reporting an LLI),

 H_1: the prevalence of LLI in the population is not 24% (written as $p \neq 0.24$)

(b) H_0: the survival rate of those on drug A is the same as that of those on drug B (written as $p_A = p_B$ where p_A is the proportion surviving on drug A and p_B is the proportion surviving on drug B),

 H_1: the survival rate of those on drug A is higher than that of those on drug B (written as $p_A > p_B$)

(c) H_0: the mean waiting time for one specialty in hospital A is the same as that in hospital B (written as $\mu_A = \mu_B$ where μ_A is the mean for hospital A and μ_B is the mean for hospital B),

 H_1: the mean waiting time for those in hospital A is different from that for hospital B (written as $\mu_A \neq \mu_B$).

Notice the difference between the first and the third examples on the one hand, and the middle example. In scenarios (a) and (c) we are not bothered about the direction of the difference under the alternative hypothesis, just that there is a difference. In scenario (b) we believe that the difference can only be in one direction. If we believe the difference can only be in one direction, e.g. that the prevalence of LLI can only be lower than expected or that one drug must be better than another, then we have a **one-tailed** test. If we believe that the difference can be in either direction, then we have a **two-tailed** test. Many commentators believe that you should always use two-tailed tests. For example, even if you are testing a new drug that should have better outcomes than an old drug, or a placebo, there is always a possibility that it will perform worse. If we just concentrated on seeing if it performed better or not (i.e. a one-tailed test), when it actually performed worse, then we would not detect that it performed worse in our test. As the situations where one-tailed tests are used are infrequent, we shall concentrate on two-tailed tests. The decision as to whether to make a one- or two-tailed test should be made before data collection. Often, only the null hypothesis is given, with the two-tailed alternative assumed.

8.3.3 Visual representation of hypothesis testing

You may be curious as to why we are using the terms one- and two-'tailed' tests. 'Sided' is another word that can replace 'tailed' and is perhaps more easy to relate to hypothesis testing.

 Let us assume that the mean waiting time for a sample of patients from a district for a particular operation is $\bar{x}$ days. Waiting times are normally distributed in this example. The population mean waiting time for the district is μ days and standard deviation is σ days for the year. Does the sample differ significantly from the district average?

Well, we can draw the distribution of our sample data based on the population mean, μ, and the population standard deviation, σ. Remember, the normal distribution is centred by the mean at zero standard deviations in Figure 8.3 and shaped by the standard deviation.

Figure 8.3

Normal distribution with shaded region being the critical region where the null hypothesis is rejected at the 95% level

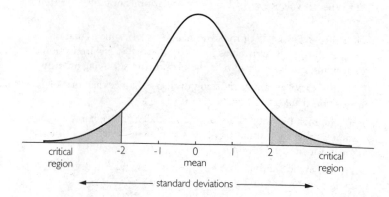

Also, remember that the area under the normal curve represents probability. This is shown in Figure 8.3. The shaded area is called the **critical region** and is in the 'tails' of the distribution on either side, i.e. the area furthest away from the centre, where the rarer values lie. If our sample mean is in this critical region then we reject the null hypothesis that the sample is the same as the district population. The critical region is often set at 5%, i.e. 2.5% of the area of the curve in each tail; this is the point 2 (or 1.96 to be exact) standard deviations away from the mean. The area in between the critical regions under the curve in Figure 8.3 represents a probability of 95%, the central 95%. This indicates that the sample mean would have to be in the outer, or extreme, 5% of the values to be regarded as different from the population mean and the difference between the sample mean and the population mean is then considered by convention as unlikely to have arisen by chance alone. If we had performed a one-tailed test (i.e. concentrated on just one of the tails of the distribution) the critical region would have covered 5% of just the one, appropriate tail, either higher or lower. The critical region does not have to be 5%, it can be 10%, 1%, 0.1%, for example. Convention alone has set it at 5%.

As you can see from the above, we do not have to prove in scenario (a) that the prevalence is exactly 24% in order to accept the null hypothesis, nor that the proportions in scenario (b) or the means in scenario (c) are exactly the same. What we do instead is to assess the evidence against the null hypothesis and try and see how unlikely it is. We can never be entirely sure but we want to assess the probability that H_0 is not true. If we can build up enough evidence against it, then we will reject H_0 in favour of H_1 **based on the evidence that we have obtained**. We assess the probability that the null hypothesis is true on the basis of our sample data. We are using the sample data to see what we can infer about the population from which we took the sample.

To accept the null hypothesis, we do not have to prove beyond all reasonable doubt that, for example, the prevalence of LLI is exactly 24%, only that the probability of it being 24% is not so small that it is extremely unlikely. Many commentators frown on saying that we accept null hypotheses. Instead they prefer to say that we 'do not reject them'. The difference is subtle but important.

This brings us to significance levels and p-values.

8.3.4 Hypothesis testing – some definitions

The **test statistic** is the statistic on which the test will be based. Examples we shall be considering include the t-test, the F-test and the chi-square statistic. Do not confuse the test statistic with our sample and population summary statistics, which refer to the mean, median, sum or proportion, for example.

The **significance** level states how much evidence against the null hypothesis we will accept as decisive; i.e. the size of the critical region. This is often denoted by α. This is the probability of rejecting the null hypothesis when it is in fact true. A significance level of 5% is the most popular and this implies that about once in every 20 occasions we will reject the null hypothesis when it is actually true. This is often called a Type I error (see section 8.6.4).

The **p-value** (also sometimes reported as the P-value) is the probability of getting a particular outcome by chance (e.g. in the process of random selection) if the null hypothesis is true. So, in scenario (a) above, if our sample statistic was a prevalence of LLI of 26%, then the p-value would be the probability of getting a prevalence of LLI of 26% or higher in the sample given that, in reality, the real figure was 24%. Similarly, if the sample figure was 15%, the p-value would be the probability of getting a prevalence of LLI of 15% or less given that, in reality, the real prevalence was 24%. The smaller the p-value, the greater the likelihood that this result was not merely due to chance.

In hypothesis testing (or significance testing as it is sometimes called), after the null and alternative hypotheses have been selected, a significance level is chosen. Then the test statistic is calculated. A computer program will also give you the p-value. The p-value can be compared to the significance level and if the p-value is smaller, then the test is significant **at this level**. If performed manually, we need to consult tables and compare our test statistic to the value in the table at our selected significance level. At the 5% significance level (where a result is said to be statistically significant if the p-value is less than 0.05) in Appendix B in the normal distribution tables, Table B2, the value is 1.96. Due to the symmetry of the normal distribution, this means we will reject the null hypothesis at the 5% level for a two-tailed test if our test statistic value lies outside the region ($-1.96, 1.96$).

If it is significant, we reject the null hypothesis at this level; if not, we do not reject the null hypothesis. A good habit to get into, instead of reporting that a result is significant at the 5% level or the 1% level or, alternatively, not significant at the 5% level or the 1% level, is to state the p-value explicitly, i.e. $p = 0.03$ or $p = 0.07$, which gives more information to the reader and allows him/her to decide on its significance.

An example of the general philosophy behind hypothesis testing will now be considered, using the Z-test, specifically for proportion testing, and move on to the more common tests in the next chapter.

8.4 THE Z-TEST

The Z-test makes use of the standard normal distribution we encountered in Chapter 6. The Z-test has the assumption that the data comes from a normal distribution and that the population variance is known; or that the sample size is large and we can apply the central limit theorem and use the sample variance to approximate the population variance. Most computer packages nowadays tend to use the t-test for comparing means between groups rather than the Z-test and we shall be exploring the t-test in the next chapter.

The Z-test is based on calculating the test statistic, z, given by the formula:

$$\frac{\text{observed value} - \text{expected value}}{\text{standard error of expected value}}$$

However, often we will not have enough information about our expected value and will need to use the standard error of the observed value as an estimate for the standard error of the expected value in order to calculate the denominator. This is the general formula for the t-test, which we shall investigate in Chapter 9.

For an example of hypothesis testing, we shall consider testing proportions based on using the central limit theorem and the Z-test. Other (parametric) tests we shall be using in Chapter 9 will have the same general principle.

8.5 PROPORTION TESTING

Remember that, when discussing the central limit theorem, we stated that for large samples we can use normal approximations for binomial distributions. In particular, the sample proportion p will be approximately normal for large sample sizes and we used this feature in our confidence interval estimation. We can use this approximation in hypothesis testing for proportions when our sample size is large.

8.5.1 Testing a sample proportion against a standard or expected proportion for the population

The standard error for a proportion is:

$$\sqrt{p(1-p)/n} \ .$$

When we want to compare a proportion picked up from a sample to an expected or standard proportion for the population we use the formula:

$$z = \frac{p - \tilde{p}}{\sqrt{\tilde{p}\,(1 - \tilde{p})/n}} \quad ,$$

where $\tilde{p}$ is our expected proportion. We are using the standard formula mentioned above and are comparing the observed value with the expected value and the denominator is the standard error of the expected value.

Let us think back to our LLI study and compare our prevalence of LLI (0.33) for people aged 18 and over with that expected from Census data (0.24). We will assume for now that our sample adequately represents the population in terms of age and sex. Our null hypothesis is that the prevalence of LLI is 0.24 (or 24%), our alternative is that it is not. We shall use a two-tailed test as we did not know before we started the study whether our sample figure would be higher or lower than expected and we shall take a significance level of 1%, to be more confident in our conclusions. Looking at the normal distribution Table B2 in Appendix B where $\alpha = 0.01$, at the 1% significance level (i.e. 100% – 99% = 1% or 0.01) the figure is 2.576. This indicates that we would not reject our null hypothesis if z is in the range (– 2.576, 2.576). Using the above equation we can enter these figures to get a value for our test statistic, z.

$$z = \frac{0.33 - 0.24}{\sqrt{(0.24 \times 0.76)\,/\,2867}} = 11.29$$

As you can see, z is comfortably outside the range for not rejecting the null hypothesis and so we can state at the 1% significance level that we reject from our data the null hypothesis that the prevalence of LLI is 24% in the study population.

Let us see what would have happened if our sample size was 100 (still large enough to justify using this normal approximation). We replace 2867 by 100 in the above formula for z, which would now equal 2.11 (please check for yourself), and we would not have rejected our null hypothesis based on this data. This does not mean the null hypothesis is right, although it may well be, it just means that we do not have enough evidence against it with our data. The smaller sample size here has meant that we can be less sure that the real prevalence of LLI is not 24% – an indicator of the influence of sample size on obtaining conclusions and why it is worth getting the sample size right. If the sample size is not large enough, you may miss significant results; unnecessarily large and you waste resources.

8.5.2 Comparing proportions between two groups

When comparing two proportions we normally test the null hypothesis that the proportions are equal and assess the evidence against the null hypothesis as before. Again, we divide the difference between the observed difference and expected difference by the standard error of the expected difference. If we assume that the first sample proportion is from population A and the second from population B then the variance of the difference between the proportions can be calculated as follows:

$$\text{Var}_{\text{dif}} = \frac{p_A(1-p_A)}{n_A} + \frac{p_B(1-p_B)}{n_B} \, .$$

We take the square root of this to find our standard error of the differences. Our expected difference is, of course, zero (no difference in the proportions) while our observed difference is $p_A - p_B$. Therefore, we have our formula for finding the Z statistic, and it is as follows:

$$z = \frac{(p_A - p_B) - 0}{\sqrt{\text{Var}_{\text{dif}}}} \, .$$

Let us compare the prevalence of LLI among males to that among females for those aged 65 and over. From Table 5.5 we can see that 170 out of 282 men aged 65 and over reported an LLI, i.e. $p_M = 0.60$ (170 divided by 282); and 264 out of 382 females reported an LLI, i.e. $p_F = 0.69$ (264 divided by 382). The variance of the difference, then, is:

$$\frac{0.60 \times 0.40}{282} + \frac{0.69 \times 0.31}{382} = 0.0014,$$

using the equation above and, therefore,

$$z = \frac{(0.60 - 0.69) - 0}{\sqrt{0.0014}} = -2.40 \, .$$

We compare this to values for the normal distribution in Table B2 in Appendix B and see that the figure at the 5% level is, again, 1.96 ($p = 0.05$) and at the 1% level is, again, 2.576 ($p = 0.01$). Therefore, our acceptance region at the 5% level is (– 1,96, 1.96) and at the 1% level is (– 2.576, 2.576). Our value for z is between these two regions, at – 2.40. We do not, therefore, reject the null hypothesis of no difference at the 1% level but reject it at the 5% level. We have evidence to suggest that there is a difference in the prevalence of LLI between men and women in our study population. Check for yourself what the result would have been if we had had the same proportions from sample sizes of 100 males and 100 females.

It is often advised that a continuity correction is made to the above formulae for both the single-proportion and two-proportion tests as we are only approximating the binomial distribution by the normal distribution. This will have little effect for large sample sizes but may change the conclusion for smaller sample sizes. For more information on this, see Altman, 1991.

A different method, with the same result, of comparing proportions between two groups will be shown in Chapter 10 when we look at the **chi-square test** for 2 × 2 tables. This is likely to be your more usual approach.

8.6 MORE ON HYPOTHESIS TESTING

The chapter so far should have given you the idea of what statistical inference is trying to achieve and should stand you in good stead when we put this into practice in the next couple of chapters. In the next chapter we shall look at statistical tests both with and without the normal distribution assumption. We shall also move on to comparing between more than two groups. You will be pleased to read that we shall try and keep away from the formulae and more on to explaining what each test does and what information a computer package is likely to give and how to interpret it. It cannot be emphasized enough that it is important for you to understand when a particular test is appropriate for your data and your needs, when it is not and what the output means that is displayed on your computer. Now that we are in the days of user-friendly computer packages in which you just need to click a button a couple of times to run the analysis rather than perform it manually with calculator and paper, more and more people are tempted to take on statistics. In some ways this is a good thing, but it runs the risk of people abusing statistics and statistical analyses.

Knowledge and understanding is the key; so, even if you are not sure how exactly the test statistic is calculated, you should understand the basis behind it, what it means and does not mean, and when it should and should not be used.

8.6.1 Back to the *p*-value and significance levels ...

In the examples in this chapter we have calculated the test statistic and compared it to values in a table based on the normal distribution. Not a *p*-value in sight. However, computer programs will give you *p*-values and it is up to you to assess their significance. A *p*-value of 0.02 is significant at the 5% level (i.e. $\alpha = 0.05$) as it is less than 0.05 but not at the 1% level (i.e. $\alpha = 0.01$). Yet how different is a *p*-value of 0.02 to a *p*-value of 0.01? One has a probability of 2 in 100 of obtaining a result more extreme than that obtained if the null hypothesis is actually true and the other has a probability of 1 in 100. You may not consider there to be much difference, in fact, between *p*-values of 0.02 and 0.01 – and you would be right. People, particularly those inexperienced with statistics, often talk about the almost Holy-Grail-like figure of a significance level of 5%, equivalent to a p-value of 0.05. A p-value of 0.04 will be considered significant and weighty conclusions will be drawn while a p-value of 0.06 will be considered insignificant and the analysis will quickly be deleted from memory. But there really is so very little difference between the two values, which is why the computer habit of giving p-values and the growing trend in reporting p-values in journals and articles is so much more helpful and informative than stating that a result is statistically significant (or not) at the 5% level. The reader can then also draw conclusions about the significance; for example, if testing a new drug, perhaps with greater side effects, against an old drug you may wish to be more certain in claiming its effectiveness and go for a 1% level rather than the conventional 5% level.

You may be curious as to why the 5% level was taken as the traditional level of significance to compare results against. Well, it was a British statistician, Sir Ronald Fisher, who suggested that this was a convenient level of significance if a cut-off point was needed and his work, at the time and 30 years and more after his death, has been greatly influential in the field of statistics. Another convention that is sometimes used is that one asterisk (*) is put alongside the result if is significant at the 5% ($p < 0.05$) level, two asterisks (**) if it significant at the 1% ($p < 0.01$) level and three asterisks (***) if it is significant at the 0.1% level ($p < 0.001$).

8.6.2 Interpreting statistical significance

If we attempted to detect a difference between two groups and we obtained a p-value of less than 0.05 (or even less than 0.0001) we still could not say for certain that there is a difference between the groups. Remember that we are talking in probabilities, not certainties. We can say that there is an extremely high probability that the two groups are not equivalent but we can never have a probability of 1 (or zero; when your computer states $p = 0.0000$ what it really means is $p < 0.0001$ – not the same thing). It is possible that we can perform the same study on the same population with a different sample and get a completely different result – although our study design should reduce the chances of this. If our sample size is too small, then we are unlikely to obtain statistical significance as our study will not have the power, even if there really is a difference. If it is too big, then some statistical tests will almost always give statistically significant results. Therefore, you need to use common sense in interpreting results before proudly proclaiming them.

For example, we may find that one drug is statistically more significant than another; but maybe by only a small amount. Clinicians may still feel just as inclined to use the (apparently) slightly inferior drug, particularly if it is much less expensive or the other drug has much worse side-effects. Perhaps one hypertensive drug reduces blood pressure slightly more than another, and is statistically significant, but clinically it makes extremely little difference. Or maybe we could show that someone with LLI scores 2 points worse on Physical Functioning than someone without LLI. It may be statistically significant but in reality it makes absolutely no difference to the comparative functioning of people with LLI and people without LLI. That is why statisticians tend to say tests are **statistically** significant and consult with others or let others decide on their practical importance.

We saw earlier that it is more informative to report the actual p-value than simply stating that a result is significant at the 5% level. When evaluating any paper or article in the media it is important to look not just at the significance of results and conclusions drawn from it by the author, but at the study design and the appropriateness of the tests and of the conclusions leading from it. Can we have faith in the results or should we treat them with scepticism? An apparently important result can hide poor design, inappropriate tests and misleading conclusions – you have been warned!

8.6.3 Confidence intervals and hypothesis testing

Most observers prefer and encourage the use of confidence intervals alongside, or even instead of, p-values as they give a better idea of the uncertainty (or precision) of the survey results. The wider the confidence interval, the less precise our survey was at estimating the population statistic.

Consider two confidence intervals for the difference between two means, say for General Health scores, between people without LLI and people with LLI. In study A we have a 95% confidence interval for the difference in the means that includes zero; say (– 10, 20). This suggests that we believe the real population difference in means is somewhere between those without LLI scoring 20 points higher and those without LLI scoring 10 points lower than those with LLI. In study B we have a 95% confidence interval that does not include zero; say, (10, 30). This suggests that we are very confident that the people without LLI have a mean score between 10 and 30 points higher than that of people with LLI. In a comparison of the means of two groups, if our hypothesis test does not reject the null hypothesis of equal population means (zero difference), then the confidence interval would include zero (no points difference). This is because the 95% confidence interval is linked to the 5% (100 – 95) significance level. In study B we can say without need to resort to a hypothesis test that there is a significant difference at the 5% level between these means. In study A, the difference is not significant at the 5% level.

In the same way, 99% confidence intervals are related to the 1% significance level and 90% confidence intervals related to the 10% significance level. The confidence level is a measure of the accuracy of the estimated difference and if it does not include zero then we can infer that on 95% (or whichever level we are using) of samples, the differences will be above zero (taking the largest mean first). Hence, it is unlikely that the means are equal.

Similarly, when considering whether a population mean equals a specified estimate, if our confidence interval for the point estimate from the sample data does not include the hypothesized figure, then we know we will reject the null hypothesis at the related significance level.

For more on the use of confidence intervals and the interpretation of confidence intervals and p-values see, for example, Altman (1996) and Greenhalgh (1997b).

8.6.4 Types of error

We have already mentioned the Type I error but we shall now return to this. Imagine a test of a null hypothesis, based on a sample, making inferences about the population from which this sample was obtained. There are four possible outcomes.

- **Outcome 1:** We do not reject the null hypothesis when it is, indeed, true – (hurrah!).

- **Outcome 2:** We reject the null hypothesis when it is, in fact, true – (boo and hiss!).

- **Outcome 3:** We reject the null hypothesis when it is, indeed, false – (hurrah again!).

- **Outcome 4:** We do not reject the null hypothesis when it is, in fact, false – (boo and hiss again!).

Outcome 2 is called a **Type I error**, a false-positive result, and the probability of this is the significance level, α. With a significance level of 5%, we only have a 5% chance of rejecting H_0 when it is really true. Outcome 4 is called a **Type II error**, a false-negative result, and the probability of this is symbolized by β. $1 - \beta$ is called the **power** and statistical tests are usually selected partially on the basis of their power to reject the null hypothesis when it is really false. We shall talk more about this when we consider parametric and non-parametric tests. The possible outcomes associated with this type of hypothesis testing are often illustrated as in Figure 8.4.

Sample sizes are calculated on the basis of their ability to detect a significant difference if there is one; hence, sample size calculations are often called power calculations. Too small a sample is likely to lead to

Figure 8.4

Possible outcomes
of hypothesis testing

		H_0 true	H_0 false
Decision	Do not reject H_0	Correct decision	Type II error
	Reject H_0	Type I error	Correct decision

a non-significant result regardless of whether there is a difference or not, hence possibly leading to a Type II error.

8.6.5 Problems with multiple testing

The problem we have with hypothesis testing is that it is all based on probabilities. We can be reasonably certain about our result and conclusion but we can never be 100% certain. If you think of the case when we set α at 5%, this, in fact, means that, on average, one in 20 tests will lead to rejecting the null hypothesis when it is really true. Good odds if you are only conducting one or two tests but if you are conducting a large number of them, known as multiple testing, then in one out of every 20 you are likely to reject the null hypothesis when you should not. One way around this problem is to use a lower significance level, say 1%; in which case we should only make Type I errors once in every 100 tests. Obviously, this would mean that we would need much stronger evidence from our sample to reject the null hypothesis. We return to this in the next chapter.

8.7 SUMMARY

In this chapter we have discussed confidence intervals and have started to look at the often baffling minefield of hypothesis testing. We have looked at the basics, including null and alternative hypotheses, types of error, significance levels, p-values and comparing the expected value with the observed value. These lie at the basis of formal statistical tests and set us up nicely for the next chapter. The importance of the normal distribution has again been highlighted, as has the lack of certainty we can place on anything (apart from being certain about this lack of certainty!). We rely on high or low probabilities. Do not get caught up in a strict 5% cut-off point trap, and use your common sense as well as statistical reasoning on your data.

In the next chapter, we expand on the statistical tests referred to here, and these will be the ones you find yourself using most

8.8 ANSWERS TO EXERCISE

For 90%, the figure for 15 DF in Table B3 in Appendix B is 1.753; therefore the 95% confidence interval is (67.25, 82.69). For 99%, the figure for 15 DF in the table is 2.947; therefore the 99% confidence interval is (61.99, 87.95).

9 COMMON APPROACHES TO STATISTICAL TESTING

9.1 INTRODUCTION

This book has been specifically designed to follow the sequence of a study, from initial 'ponderings' through survey design, starting to look at and describe the data, and now to more formal statistical tests. This 'testing' is what many people understand as 'what statistics is all about', whereas summarizing and describing data and presentation of confidence intervals is the more important part of statistics for many health service researchers.

However, tests do have their place, and in this chapter we shall start by comparing two groups on one interval- or ratio-measured variable and continue on to comparing more than two groups and more than one variable. We shall assess the use of both parametric tests and their non-parametric equivalents.

9.2 PARAMETRIC AND NON-PARAMETRIC TESTS

What is the point of the central limit theorem and of worrying about the assumptions that underlie data handling? Why not just go for a test that has no assumptions about the underlying distribution (known as a non-parametric test or, sometimes, a distribution-free test)? Well, there are a number of reasons for preferring to use parametric tests if we can meet the assumptions behind them. Firstly, they are more powerful. That is, they are more likely to detect a significant difference (i.e. reject the null hypothesis) if there really is one than their non-parametric counterparts. Secondly, non-parametric tests are often based on ranking of values rather than on the actual values themselves, and are used for skewed data, for example. One consequence of this is that non-parametric tests use less of the data than their parametric equivalents. It is also harder to produce estimates and related confidence intervals of relevant statistics using non-parametric tests. There is not much point in reporting the mean and standard deviation if our analysis is going to be based on ranks, and it is difficult to get any meaningful measure of rankings. Normally, in non-parametric analysis, the median is given and it is possible to produce a confidence interval for the median (see, for example, Altman, 1991). Final disadvantages of non-parametric analysis are that the type of analysis is limited and that they are less commonly used and, therefore, not recognized by many as appropriate for their situation or understood when performed.

9.3 COMPARISON BETWEEN TWO INDEPENDENT GROUPS ON ONE VARIABLE

9.3.1 The *t*-test for two independent samples

Consider the situation where you wish to compare the means of an interval/ratio variable between two independent groups. For example, we may wish to see if males and females score similarly on the Physical Functioning (PF) scale or whether those with limiting long-term illness tend to be younger or older than those without LLI. Our null hypotheses would in the first case be that the mean PF scale score is the same for both males and females and in the second case that the mean age is the same for the LLI and non-LLI groups.

The common approach to such a comparison is to use the *t*-test. This is applicable when the population variances are unknown and they are estimated using the sample variances, but we believe that the data is drawn from normal distributions or the sample sizes are large and we can exploit the central limit theorem. The *t*-test uses values from a distribution called the *t*-distribution, rather than the normal distribution. For large sample sizes the results are virtually identical to a Z-test. This is because, as the sample size increases, the *t*-distribution gets ever closer to the normal distribution that is used by the Z-test. Compare tables B2 and B3 in Appendix B and see how close the figures in the *t*-distribution table get to the related figures (i.e. at the same α) in the normal distribution table as you move down the page to ∞ degrees of freedom.

The *t*-distribution was devised in 1908 by William S. Gossett. Because of his wish for anonymity he published under the name 'Student' and, hence, Student's *t*-distribution and Student's *t*-test (to give them their full names) arrived. The two-sample *t*-test is sometimes known as the independent samples *t*-test.

The assessment of the equality of the population variances from which the two groups are taken is important in deciding which of the two 'flavours' of the two-sample *t*-test is most appropriate. One is for when we assume that the two groups have equal variances and the other for when they have unequal variances. The difference is important as using the equal variance *t*-test when the variances are unequal may, on some occasions, lead to incorrect *p*-values. However, using the unequal variance *t*-test when the population variances are equal will sometimes lead to *p*-values higher than they would otherwise be. We shall consider the differences between the two when we look at an example, shortly.

SPSS for Windows calculates both *t*-test statistics and also gives you the result of the Levene test, which tests the null hypothesis that the population variances of the two groups are equal. This is shown in Table 9.1, which we will examine shortly. MINITAB will also perform the Levene test and allows you to decide on whether to use the equal or unequal variance version of the *t*-test.

It is quite possible (and straightforward) to calculate *t*-tests manually and until a few years ago you would have had to use calculators at least. However, for large sample sizes it would get pretty tedious calculating the means and standard deviations and so we assume you would normally use a computer package to produce these tests.

However, we will start by performing the two-sample t-test manually; then move on to explaining the output from SPSS for Windows t-test calculation. We will use a simple example to demonstrate how to calculate the two-sample t-test for small sample sizes. Imagine a study of two groups. In this example, a doctor in a general practice is undecided between two forms of diet. Diet 1 involves a general education on the best foods to eat while diet 2 is a strict diet by which the senior partner in the practice swears. The doctor uses a random numbers table to allocate the 20 dieters he saw in one week to one of the two diets for his small study. He ends up with 11 on diet 1 and nine on diet 2. After a set period of time he records the success of the diet in terms of pounds lost as shown below (we shall assume that those on diet 2 followed it exactly and that other characteristics, like amount of exercise, are similar in both groups).

$$\text{Diet 1:} \quad 2 \quad 9 \quad 4 \quad 8 \quad 6 \quad 9 \quad 2 \quad 4 \quad 3 \quad 7 \quad 5$$
$$\text{Diet 2:} \quad 3 \quad 10 \quad 9 \quad 7 \quad 6 \quad 12 \quad 8 \quad 5 \quad 4$$

Assuming that this data is drawn from populations in which weight loss is normally distributed, we can conduct a two-sample t-test. We use the evidence from this study to see what we can infer about the two diets in general. The null hypothesis is that the mean weight loss is the same on both diets. The alternative hypothesis is that they are not the same, that one diet gives a greater weight loss. We are not saying which diet we are looking to give a greater loss, so we have a two-tailed test.

Calculate, first of all, the mean and standard deviations for the two groups. Remember, we are estimating the population mean and standard deviation based on the sample data so the denominator for the standard deviation formula will be $n - 1$ rather than n (see Chapter 6 if you are not quite sure what we are on about here). You should get:

Diet 1: mean $(\bar{x}_1)$ 5.364   SD (s_1) 2.6181 $n_1 = 11$;
Diet 2: mean $(\bar{x}_2)$ 7.111   SD (s_2) 2.9345 $n_2 = 9$.

The first thing we need to do is to calculate the standard error of the difference in the means using what is called the pooled variance approach, which assumes equality of the two population variances. The formula for the standard error of the difference of the means for equal variances is:

$$SE_{dif} = \sqrt{\frac{(n_1 - 1)s_1^2 + (n_2 - 1)s_2^2}{n_1 + n_2 - 2}} \times \sqrt{\frac{1}{n_1} + \frac{1}{n_2}} \quad .$$

The part in the first square root is the pooled variance and the square root gives the pooled standard deviation. This is basically the average of the two group standard deviations but weighted by the size of the groups. To get the standard error of the differences we multiply it by the second part. Normally, of course, this would be calculated by the computer.

Using our example data we get:

$$SE_{dif} = \sqrt{\frac{(10 \times 2.6181^2) + (8 \times 29345^2)}{11 + 9 - 2}} \times \sqrt{\frac{1}{11} + \frac{1}{9}}$$

If you work that out it gives you a standard error of the difference of the means equal to 1.2420. This is needed in order to calculate the t-statistic, which is done using a familiar formula:

$$\frac{\text{observed difference in means} - \text{expected difference in means}}{\text{standard error of observed difference}}$$

Our expected difference, if we are assessing the equality of the population means, will be zero, i.e. we expect the two diets to result in the same amount of weight loss. Remember, we are using the observed data to estimate the population data. Hence the denominator is the standard error of the observed difference rather than the expected difference (as we do not know this standard error).

This gives us in symbols, the equation:

$$t = \frac{(\bar{x}_1 - \bar{x}_2) - 0}{SE_{dif}} \, ,$$

where t is our test statistic. We compare the means for diet 1 and diet 2, subtract our expected difference (normally zero) and divide by our previously calculated standard error of the difference in the means. Inserting our figures gives us a value for t of $(5.364 - 7.111) / 1.2420 = -1.41$.

We need to compare this figure of -1.41 with the figure at the 5% significance level in the t-distribution, shown in Table B3 in Appendix B, to see if we reject our null hypothesis or not.

The number of degrees of freedom for the two-sample t-test is calculated by adding the sizes of the two groups and subtracting 2 (in symbols, $n_1 + n_2 - 2$) and so we compare our t-statistic with the figures in Table B3 in Appendix B on the row for 11 + 9 - 2 or 18 degrees of freedom. The symmetry of the t-distribution (as with the normal distribution) means that we can remove the minus sign from our t-statistic and compare 1.41 with the figure in the table where $\alpha = 0.05$ (i.e. a 5% level of significance, two-tailed) which is 2.101. As 1.41 is less than 2.101, the p-value must be greater than 0.05 (the smaller the p-value, the larger the test statistic) so we cannot reject the null hypothesis of equal weight loss at the 5% level. Based on our evidence, therefore, we cannot say that one of the diets causes more weight loss than the other. If the t-statistic had been greater than 2.101, or less than -2.101, we would have rejected the null hypothesis of equal weight loss at the 5% level and have reasonable evidence that one diet (diet 2, since it has the largest mean weight loss) leads to a greater weight loss.

You will be pleased to know that, after calculating these figures by hand and calculator, a statistical package gave the same result. The computer gave a p-value of 0.176.

While we had no reason to believe that the population variances were different (and we could test it formally), what if we had decided to be ultra-cautious and use the unequal variances version of the t-test? This also has the null hypothesis that the population means are equal, i.e. the diets lead to equal weight loss, and the alternative hypothesis that they are not equal. We replace that complicated formula for the standard error of the difference of the means in the formula for the t-statistic by the rather more simpler formula of:

$$\sqrt{\frac{s_1^2}{n_1} + \frac{s_2^2}{n_2}} \ .$$

The degrees of freedom, however, are much more complicated to work out and we will not overburden you with the method, other than to say that the degrees of freedom will now be smaller and that this will make it more difficult to detect a significant difference. So if we have no reason to believe that the population variances are different we should use the equal variances version, certainly for small sample sizes, where the difference between the two versions is more marked.

The resulting test statistic using our new calculation for the standard error of the differences is -1.39. Again, this is less than 2.101 so we do not reject the null hypothesis at the 5% significance level.

The actual p-value is 0.186 (calculated by computer). As you can see this is slightly higher than that for the equal variances test; this will usually be the case when the population variances are equal. For large sample sizes, the two statistics will actually be very similar.

9.3.2 A further example

Let us use an example based on a higher sample size than that in our above example. Here we have hypothesized about the differences in General Health scores on the Short Form-36 between those who are currently married and those who are not (i.e. combining the single with the separated/divorced and the widowed). We saw from Chapter 6 that there was an obvious difference between those reporting a limiting long-term illness and those not reporting an LLI in their GH scores, but perhaps marital status is also a factor in poor general health. Does being married improve health (perhaps due to companionship and reduced loneliness) or is it linked to poorer health? The computer output is shown in Table 9.1 for *t*-tests within both the LLI and non-LLI groups, comparing the married group with the non-married group.

Reported LLI

t-tests for Independent Samples of MARITAL   marital status

Variable	Number of Cases	Mean	SD	SE of Mean
GH general health				
Not married	180	42.4032	21.597	1.610
Married	380	47.1792	23.144	1.187

Mean Difference = −4.7759
Levene's Test for Equality of Variances: *F* = 1.860   *P* = 0.173
t-test for Equality of Means

Variances	*t*-value	df	2-Tail Sig	SE of Diff	95% CI for Diff
Equal	−2.33	558	0.020	2.050	(−8.803, −0.749)
Unequal	−2.39	374.39	0.017	2.000	(−8.709, −0.843)

No LLI

t-tests for Independent Samples of MARITAL   marital status

Variable	Number of Cases	Mean	SD	SE of Mean
GH general health				
Not married	136	76.0980	16.789	1.140
Married	434	74.5409	17.826	0.856

Mean Difference = −1.5571
Levene's Test for Equality of Variances: *F* = 0.097   *P* = 0.755
t-test for Equality of Means

Variances	*t*-value	df	2-Tail Sig	SE of Diff	95% CI for Diff
Equal	0.90	568	0.368	1.728	(−1.837, 4.951)
Unequal	0.93	237.97	0.353	1.675	(−1.742, 4.856)

Let us start with the LLI group, the top half of Table 9.1. SPSS for Windows calls the two-sample *t*-test '*t*-tests for independent samples'. '*Marital*' is the name we have given to the variable that states whether a respondent is married or not. In the top of the table you are given general descriptive data of the two groups. There are 180 respondents who are not married and 380 who are married (there were also some people who did not answer the question on marital status but these were few – 43, about 7% – so we shall ignore them; we do not believe their answers would have affected our results).

The mean GH score for the not married group is 42.4032 and for the married group is 47.1792. This gives us a sample mean difference of – 4.7759, but can we say with any confidence that there is a difference in the population means based on this sample data? The standard deviations ('SD') are given, as are the standard errors of the means ('SE of Mean'); check for yourselves that the standard errors of the means are the standard deviations divided by the square roots of the sample sizes.

The next thing we have is the test for the equality of the population variances using 'Levene's test for equality of variances' to see if we have any reason to worry about using the equal variances approach to the t-test. The Levene test has the null hypothesis that the population variances are equal and the alternative hypothesis that they are not equal. As you can see, this gives an F-statistic. However, interpretation of the associated p-value is the same as ever and there is an associated p-value of 0.173. This p-value is greater than 0.05 (the 5% significance level) and even 0.10 (the 10% significance level) so we have no reason to dispute the equality of the population variances. We do not reject the null hypothesis of equal population variances and so we shall concentrate on that version of the t-test.

In the bottom table for the LLI group we can read the top line for 'equal' variances. The t-value is the t-statistic, as we calculated in the previous example. 'df' is the degrees of freedom, which for equal variances, remember, equate to $n_1 + n_2 - 2$ or $180 + 380 - 2$, which equals 558 (notice the different number of degrees of freedom for the 'unequal' variances). These sample sizes are so large that the t-distribution now equates the normal distribution. The '2-Tail Sig' or p-value, is 0.020 so we can reject the null hypothesis of equal means at the 5% level, but not at the 1% level (as p is less than 0.05 but greater than 0.01). Note the similarity in 't-values' and p-values because of the large sample sizes between the equal and unequal variances calculations.

The standard error of the difference of the means ('SE of Diff') is also given. You could use the above formulas in section 9.3.1 and the data in the top part of Table 9.1 to check the results for the standard error of the difference of the means if you want. The t-value given, as you should recognize, is simply – 4.7759 divided by 2.050. Then, if you look at the bottom row (i.e. the row for large number of degrees of freedom, labelled ∞) in the t-distribution table in Table B3 in Appendix B you can see that a value of 2.33 is equivalent to a significance level of 0.02. This is the '2-Tail Sig.' stated in Table 9.1; this is, in fact, the p-value.

The last part of the table gives the 95% confidence interval for the difference in the means (remember we talked about confidence intervals in the previous chapter). We expect that the population mean difference between non-married and married GH scores is somewhere between – 0.749 and – 8.803. That is, we expect the married mean score in the population to be anywhere between 0.75 and 8.80 higher than the non-married mean score. As it does not include the value zero, then this would be a hint that we would get a significant result at the 5% level.

It seems that being married does improve your GH scores, at least for those reporting an LLI with similar characteristics to our sample. We might, however, want to look for confounding variables such as the married group perhaps being younger, which might help to explain our result. It might not be the fact of being married that reduces scores but some other variable that is highly associated with being married. We could produce a t-test to assess the age difference between the married and non-married groups. However, we shall shortly look at ways of including a number of variables in an analysis.

Now read through the table for the non-LLI group. Notice again that we have no reason to believe that the population variances are not equal but, this time, we do not have enough evidence against the null hypothesis to say that the population mean GH scores are different. Notice that the 95% confidence interval for the difference in means now includes zero.

9.3.3 The non-parametric alternative to the two-sample *t*-test

What if our data looked as if it was not from a normal distribution and the sample size was not large. Perhaps we produced a histogram that was skewed rather than the normal shape described in Chapter 6. Or maybe the sample size is small and we are using data that is commonly known to be non-normal; income, for example, where there are a few earners (outliers) who earn many times what the great majority of people do. We need to be more cautious and use a non-parametric test.

The non-parametric equivalent of the two-sample *t*-test is called the **Mann–Whitney *U* Test**. Actually, there are two derivations of this test, the one due to the combination of Mann and Whitney and one down to Wilcoxon. The test is normally called the Mann–Whitney test (not out of spite to Wilcoxon, but to avoid confusion with the Wilcoxon non-parametric alternative for paired data – see section 9.4.2). Some people go the whole hog and call what we shall call the Mann–Whitney test the Mann–Whitney–Wilcoxon test (or the Wilcoxon–Mann–Whitney test).

The Mann–Whitney test is based on the ranking of the values rather than the values themselves. Both groups are combined into one, with the values ranked in order of size irrespective of which group they are from. Remember, the *t*-test is based on comparing the mean value of the two groups. After the ranking is done, the sum of the ranks for each group is calculated. If the groups are similar, then the mean ranks for each group should be similar. The test statistic, *U*, is then calculated based on the null hypothesis that two independent groups have been drawn from the same population. *U* is used for the Mann–Whitney version – be warned, the Wilcoxon version has test statistic *W*. Special tables for the Mann–Whitney test give the relevant level of significance or, for large sample sizes, an approximation to the normal distribution is used.

The Mann–Whitney test is appropriate for data measured on at least an ordinal scale. Although it is not as powerful as the *t*-test when the *t*-test can be properly applied to the data, it is a fine alternative when there are worries about the assumptions needed for the two-sample *t*-test.

To give you an idea of how the Mann–Whitney test works, we shall look at how we would go about starting to calculate the Mann–Whitney test. Let us imagine that a small group of medical students, all rated of similar ability based on previous work, are taught a subject and split into two groups, one taught by a traditional approach for 2 hours and one by a more modern approach for 2 hours. They are then tested to see which method was most productive. The null hypothesis being that both methods are equally effective.

The marks in the test (out of 50) are below:

Traditional group (A):   42 33 27 49 41
Modern group (B):   32 38 46 17 38 26

First we need to rank the values regardless of the method by which they were taught, from smallest to largest.

Score	17	26	27	32	33	38	38	41	42	46	49
Method	B	B	A	B	A	B	B	A	A	B	A
Ranking	1	2	3	4	5	6.5	6.5	8	9	10	11

Notice that ties are given the **mean** of those ranks. Hence, the two scoring 38 are given 6.5, the mean of 6 and 7. The sum of the rankings for A is 36 (3 + 5 + 8 + 9 + 11) and for B it is 30. The mean rank for A is 7.2 (36 / 5) and for B it is 5 (30 / 6). If the two groups are similar, then the mean ranks would be similar. The Mann–Whitney statistic U is based on the number of times a value in the first group is ranked before a value in the second group. If you like, you can look at it as all the possible pairs containing one member from each group where the group A value is ranked before the group B value. The calculation of U is shown in Table 9.2.

Table 9.2

Calculation of the Mann–Whitney U statistic

A	B	Mann–Whitney U statistic
49		0
	46	
42		1
41		1
	38	
	38	
33		3
	32	
27		4
	26	
	17	
		Total = 9

In the above situation, score 49, which is the highest value and hence highest ranked, is before no B values; (0), scores 42 and 41 (the next highest group A values) are both before one B value; (1) and (1), score 33 is before three B values; (3) and score 27 is before four B values; (4). Now add the values in brackets to get $U = 0 + 1 + 1 + 3 + 4 = 9$.

Tables based on the two group sizes and the value for U are then read to obtain the significance level. If the two groups are the same in their distribution, neither of the groups should consistently be in front of values in the other group.

Wilcoxon's version gives a test statistic, which is denoted by W. W is simply the sum of the ranks in the smaller group. Hence, W in our example equals 36. Again, tables of probabilities can be read based on sample sizes and W to find the significance level but we shall assume (as is most likely) that you are using a computer. The Mann–Whitney and the Wilcoxon versions will give the same p-values. For large sample size, normal distribution approximations are taken (see Altman, 1991 for more details).

Using a computer and statistical package, we find that our test result is not significant at the 5% level as we have a p-value of 0.32. We cannot reject the null hypothesis that the two distributions are equal; i.e. we have no evidence to say that there is a difference in the two methods.

Let us see how the Wilcoxon–Mann–Whitney test fared with our example we used for the LLI study to look at the effect on General Health scores of being married or not. Table 9.3 shows the results.

We have both the Mann–Whitney test statistic (U) and the Wilcoxon test statistic (W). Both tests allow a correction for ties, i.e. where one or more values are the same. This is particularly important when the values are in different groups (for more on the problems with tied ranks see Siegal and Castellan, 1988).

Table 9.3

Mann–Whitney tests for General Health scores by marital status

LLI: 1   yes

Mann–Whitney U – Wilcoxon Rank Sum W Test

GH   general health

by   MARITAL   marital status

Mean Rank	Cases		
258.06	180	MARITAL = 1	not married
291.13	380	MARITAL = 2	married
	560	Total	

Corrected for ties

U	W	Z	2-Tailed P
30161.0	46451.0	−2.2618	0.0237

LLI: 0   no

Mann–Whitney U – Wilcoxon Rank Sum W Test

GH   general health

by   MARITAL   marital status

Mean Rank	Cases		
294.00	136	MARITAL = 1	not married
282.84	434	MARITAL = 2	married
	570	Total	

Corrected for ties

U	W	Z	2-Tailed P
28356.0	39984.0	−0.6917	0.4891

'*U*' and '*W*' give us the Mann–Whitney and Wilcoxon test statistics, respectively. The Z statistic is the normal approximation used when the sample size is large, together with the associated *p*-value (labelled '2-Tailed P' here). For sample sizes under 30, SPSS for Windows also gives an exact probability, i.e. not based on a normal distribution approximation. This non-parametric test gives the same conclusions as its parametric counterpart. In the top half of the table for the LLI group we have a *p*-value of 0.0237, so we reject the null hypothesis that marital status has no effect on General Health score at the 5% significance level. Notice that the *p*-value is very similar to that of the equal variances *t*-test.

In Table 9.3, for the LLI group, the mean ranks are calculated based on ranking all 560 cases from 1 to 560 based on score and calculating the mean of the ranks for the 180 not married people and then the mean of the ranks for the 380 married people.

9.4 COMPARISON BETWEEN TWO MATCHED GROUPS

We have just been discussing the parametric and non-parametric alternative for the case where we want to investigate the difference between two independent groups. Now we move on to discuss the case where the groups are **matched**.

The most obvious form of matching is the before and after example, i.e. a score before an intervention compared to the score after the intervention for each individual. That means the individual will have one score in the 'before' group and one score in the 'after' group, which will be matched with each other. We would expect that the before and after scores are highly correlated.

It does not have to be two scores for one individual that are matched. In case-control studies, each case is matched as closely as possible to a control on what are considered possible confounding factors such as age, sex, height, weight, and so on, depending on the study concerned. Often the case and controls may be related in some way, e.g. in studies of twins or marital couples.

9.4.1 The paired *t*-test

For the paired *t*-test to be appropriate, the study must have each member of the first group matched with one member of the other group, and from this the difference between the two scores in the pairing are calculated.

In the paired *t*-test we are interested in the difference within the pairs and hence each pair can be regarded as one subject in a single sample study. What is important is the variability within the pairing (e.g. between the before and after scores for each individual) rather than differences between the subjects in each group, which are crucial for the independent (or two) sample *t*-test. We calculate the mean and variance of the pair differences and the form of the test removes the effect of between subject variation. The assumption of the paired *t*-test is that the differences must have an approximately normal distribution, rather than that each group's data is normally distributed.

Let us pretend that we used the SF-36 as part of a before and after study with a particular kind of intervention. The question of the use of the SF-36 as an outcome tool like this is debatable and has, indeed, been debated but let us assume that it will give important and valid results. The data for one of the scales, General Health, is given in Table 9.4 along with the difference between the before and after scores for each pairing; we shall assume that the differences are normally distributed. Shortly, we shall compare the results for the paired t-test with that of its non-parametric equivalents.

Subject	Before	After	Difference
1	62	67	5
2	37	37	0
3	37	47	10
4	87	87	0
5	15	25	10
6	92	87	−5
7	67	72	5
8	72	87	15
9	62	72	10
10	87	100	13
11	25	33.33	8.33
12	57	57	0
13	87	72	−15
14	33.33	47	13.67
15	47	62	15
16	45	47	2
17	67	72	5
18	47	45	−2
19	62	72	10
20	15	25	10
21	40	45	5
22	40	47	7
23	82	72	−10
Mean	55.014	59.884	4.870
St.dev.	23.153	20.812	7.795

Table 9.4

Before and after intervention scores on the SF-36 General Health scale

Check our calculations for the mean and standard deviation of the before, after and difference scores yourself.

You will not be surprised to know now that the calculation of the test statistic is based on the formula given in section 8.4. The usual null hypothesis (as ours is here) is that there is no difference between the before and after scores; hence, the expected difference is zero. The alternative hypothesis is that there will be a difference. We might expect that the intervention will improve the scores but as we cannot be certain at the start of the study we shall stick with the two-tailed test. The calculation of the paired t-statistic is defined by:

$$\frac{\text{mean difference} - 0}{\text{standard error of the mean difference}},$$

or in symbols:

$$t = \frac{\bar{d} - 0}{s_{dif} / \sqrt{n}},$$

where $\bar{d}$ is the mean difference, s_{dif} is the standard deviation of the difference and n is, as ever, the sample size.

The other thing we have to worry about is the degrees of freedom. In the case of the paired t-test it is simply calculated as the number of pairs minus 1. In our case, therefore, we have 22 degrees of freedom.

Let us work out the t-statistic using our calculations for mean and standard deviation of the differences:

$$t = \frac{4.870}{7.795 / \sqrt{23}} = 2.996.$$

We can look at the table of the t-distribution in Table B3 in Appendix B and look along the row for degrees of freedom equal to 22. The value where $\alpha = 0.05$ is 2.074. In actual fact, if we move along the table, we can see that the value 2.996 is somewhere between $\alpha = 0.01$ and $\alpha = 0.001$ and so we can say that this result is significant at the 1% level ($p < 0.01$). Hence, we reject the null hypothesis that the before and after scores are equal at the 1% level of significance. On the basis of our evidence, we can say that the intervention has improved scores. However, although we can say that there is statistical significance in the change in SF-36 scores, we must leave it to clinicians and to the patients themselves to say whether this is an important change in their health.

Now consider the computer output for this example, shown in Table 9.5.

It is at least reassuring that we got the result right. The top part of the table gives the details for the two groups; the before scores and the after scores. 'Corr' stands for correlation and we shall not bother with

Table 9.5

Paired t-test comparing before intervention and after intervention General Health scores

t-test for Paired Samples

Variable	Number of pairs	Corr	2-tail Sig	Mean	SD	SE of Mean
BEFORE				55.0145	23.153	4.828
	23	0.943	0.000			
AFTER				59.8839	20.812	4.340

Paired Differences

Mean	SD	SE of Mean	t-value	df	2-tail Sig
−4.8694	7.795	1.625	−3.00	22	0.007

95% CI (−8.240, −1.499)

this and its related '2-tail sig' (*p*-value) until the next chapter. You should know by now that the standard error of the mean is simply the standard deviation divided by the square root of the sample size. The bottom part of the table confirms our test results. SPSS for Windows has taken the after scores from the before scores rather than the before scores from the after scores as we did, hence the figures for the mean and '*t*-value' are the negative of ours but it makes no difference. The *p*-value, described as '2-tail Sig', associated with this data the computer gives as 0.007 (as we said, between 0.01 and 0.001). The last line is also interesting. This gives the 95% confidence interval for the mean difference. As this range does not include zero then, if you remember what we said in the last chapter, this tells us that the test would be significant at the 5% level.

9.4.2 The non-parametric equivalents to the paired *t*-test

There are two commonly used equivalents to the paired *t*-test, which can be used when we are uncertain whether the differences are normally distributed and our sample size is small. Like all non-parametric tests, these are less powerful than their parametric equivalent.

These tests are called the sign test and the Wilcoxon matched pairs test. The sign test is the simplest and, probably, the oldest of all non-parametric tests and simply uses the number of positive differences in the pairings, the number of negative differences and the number of ties (i.e. zero differences). The Wilcoxon matched pairs test (or the Wilcoxon matched pairs signed rank sum test to give it its full title) extends this idea to look at the size of the difference as well as the direction of the difference and then ranks the differences in order of size (ignoring the direction). This is similar to the Mann–Whitney test except that we rank the differences ignoring direction (positive or negative), rather than the values ignoring group as we did for the Mann–Whitney test. The Wilcoxon matched pairs test is more powerful than the sign test but has more assumptions, as will be shown later. Interested readers should consult, for example, Siegal and Castellan, 1988 for further details of the calculations involved but for now we shall concentrate on the SPSS for Windows output for these two tests for our example used in the paired *t*-test.

Table 9.6 shows the results of the two tests.

The sign test's only assumption is that the data is of at least ordinal scale. The sign test shows that there were four occasions when the after score was less than the before score, 16 where the after score was greater than the before score and three where the scores were the same.

The sign test has the null hypothesis that the number of positive and negative differences are the same, i.e. that the probability of a positive difference is equal to the probability of a negative difference. This can be interpreted as follows: that the probability of randomly drawing a subject from the population whose before-intervention score is greater than their after-intervention score is 0.5, or a half, with the same probability of it being smaller. It uses the binomial distribution,

Table 9.6	Sign Test

Sign test and Wilcoxon matched pairs test for before intervention and after intervention General Health scores

Sign Test
    BEFORE
with AFTER

	Cases	
	4 − Diffs (AFTER LT BEFORE)	
	16 + Diffs (AFTER GT BEFORE)	(Binomial)
	3 Ties	2-Tailed P = 0.0118
	23 Total	

Wilcoxon Matched-Pairs Signed-Ranks Test
    BEFORE
with AFTER

Mean Rank	Cases
9.50	4 − Ranks (AFTER LT BEFORE)
10.75	16 + Ranks (AFTER GT BEFORE)
	3 Ties (AFTER EQ BEFORE)
	23 Total
Z = 2.5013	2-Tailed P = 0.0124

which gives the probability of a dichotomous outcome (i.e. outcome with only two possibilities) to calculate the p-value.

Notice that the p-value is slightly higher than that of the paired t-test but is still significant at the 5% level. The sign test is rarely applied as it uses so little of the data.

As stated earlier, the Wilcoxon matched pairs test ranks the differences between the pairs, ignoring the sign. Under the null hypothesis, the sum of the ranks for positive differences should be equal to the sum of the ranks for the negative differences.

The assumptions of the Wilcoxon matched-pairs test are, firstly, that the data is at least of ordinal scale and that the differences between pairs of observations should be on an interval/ratio scale. Secondly, the distribution of the differences should be symmetrical in nature, about the median difference. This means that if you were to draw a histogram of the differences it would be reasonably symmetrical.

The results of the Wilcoxon matched pairs test give the mean rank for the two directions. The 23 differences are ranked from 1–23 on the basis of size with direction ignored and the mean rank calculated for the two possible directions of difference. For large samples (perhaps 25–30 or more) the test statistic has an approximately normal distribution and so normal distribution tables can be used, i.e. by virtue of the central limit theorem. For small sample sizes, special probability tables are available. Notice again the slightly higher p-value. Here, however, we still reject the null hypothesis that the before and after intervention scores are equal, at the 5% level.

9.5 TESTING WHETHER A SAMPLE COMES FROM A POPULATION WITH A SPECIFIED MEAN

We may wish to assess whether our sample data has been collected from a population that we hypothesize has a particular mean. For example, consider our dieters in the example introduced in section 9.3.1. Let us say that an expert who advocates diet 1 claims than the mean weight loss on this diet is 7 lb. Does the data support this claim? Well, the t-statistic is calculated as below, from our general formula:

$$t = \frac{\text{sample mean} - \text{hypothesized mean}}{\text{standard error of sample mean}} \quad ,$$

or, in symbols:

$$t = \frac{\bar{x} - x_0}{SE} \quad ,$$

where x_0 is the hypothesized mean. We shall assume that the assumptions of the t-test are met. The null hypothesis is that the population mean diet 1 weight loss is 7 lb. The alternative hypothesis is that it is not 7 lb.

In this case:

$$t = \frac{5.364 - 7}{2.6181 / \sqrt{11}} = -2.072.$$

We have $n - 1$ degrees of freedom, which gives us 10 degrees of freedom. Again, because of the symmetry of the t-distribution we can ignore the negative sign. Study of Table B3 in Appendix B shows that $p > 0.05$ (the value at 10 degrees of freedom and $\alpha = 0.05$ is 2.228, greater than 2.072) and so we do not reject the null hypothesis that the mean weight loss is 7 lb at the 5% significance level. We cannot say that the mean weight loss from this diet is not 7 lb based on our data. The actual value of p (from computer calculations) is 0.065. This value is only slightly above 0.05 and as we do not want to get sucked into the trap of having a very strict cut-off point for significance of 0.05 as we discussed in Chapter 8, it is best anyway to report the p-value exactly.

9.6 MORE GROUPS, MORE VARIABLES

You are probably sitting there, sinking your fourth gin and tonic or sipping on your hot cocoa, thinking that this is all very well but what if we have three groups, or four, or more than one variable? We have already warned you against multiple testing and you have probably gathered by now that producing many *t*-tests for each pair of groups on each variable is not the way to go. However, fear not, for there are ways around this problem. We are about to enter the world of the **ANOVA** – or ANalysis Of VAriance.

We will discuss the simpler form of the ANOVA in some detail and give general descriptions of the more complicated forms. In the world of computerized statistical packages, understanding when a test is appropriate and when it is not, and what it means and what the results mean is more important than the rudiments of how it is calculated. However, we suggest that for the more complicated forms of analysis you seek expert advice and/or follow the further reading.

9.6.1 More than two groups

We shall start by considering what we would do if we wanted to assess the difference between more than two independent groups on one variable. For example, we might want to compare the General Health scale scores between people with musculoskeletal-type LLIs, mental-type LLIs and respiratory-type LLIs, or compare length of waiting list of people for one specialty in four different hospitals.

The parametric test for this situation is the analysis of variance, or ANOVA. This has been attributed to Sir Ronald Fisher, who also developed the *F*-distribution, which is used in ANOVA and was named after him. If you like, you can consider this the extension of the two-sample *t*-test.

There are a number of different forms of the ANOVA, depending on the type of analysis and numbers of independent variables. We shall start, however, as is traditional, with the simplest form and work our way up. Here, as for the *t*-test, we have a categorical independent variable, except now it can have two or more categories or groups – e.g. a group reporting limiting long-term illness and a group who do not, or marital status (broken down into married, single, divorced/separated and widowed groups) – and a continuous or discrete dependent variable – e.g. score on the General Health scale. In the **one-way ANOVA** we simply assess differences between groups based on one independent variable.

The ANOVA looks at variability both within groups and between groups. The test is the **F-test** and the test statistic is the **F-statistic**, based on the aforementioned **F-distribution**. The idea is that not only will you have variability between the groups but you will also have variability within each of the groups. Just because a number of people report an LLI does not mean that they are all the same or that they will all score similarly on the General Health scale. The *F*-statistic tests to see how large the variability is between the groups as compared to the size of the variability within each group. The *F*-statistic is also known, in a more descriptive manner, as the **F-ratio**. This is because the F-statistic is basically the ratio of the variance between groups to the variance within groups. The variance between groups is known as the explained variance because it is the variance in the dependent variable that is accounted for by the variance in the independent variable, i.e. the result of being in one group rather than another – for example, of having an LLI. The variance within groups is known as the **unexplained** or **error variance**.

The assumptions behind the test are similar to the *t*-test in that the underlying population distribution should be normal and the population variances of the groups should be equal. The Levene test is again on hand to test for the equality of variance.

It is perhaps easiest to study an ANOVA table to describe more about how the one-way ANOVA works. The general practice in which we carried out the study has a boundary that stretches across five electoral wards; so one question is to what extent there are differences between the wards, or 'locality' as we have labelled the relevant variable. Again, we have produced two tests: one for those who reported an LLI and one for those who did not. The results are produced in Table 9.7.

The null hypothesis is that all the group (i.e. ward) means are equal. The alternative hypothesis is that they are not equal. Note that we are not trying to say which of the locality means might be the largest or smallest; nor are we saying which is or are different from the rest. For the LLI group, in the top half of Table 9.7, looking at the descriptive statistics, we might feel that group (in this case, ward) 4 has a smaller GH mean score than group 1 but this should not concern us for the moment.

You should now quickly understand all of the descriptive statistics by now. If not, go back through the relevant sections of text before you proceed.

Levene's test for homogeneity of variances has the null hypothesis that the population variances are equal. The '2-tail Sig' for the LLI group suggests that this may not be the case and we should not accept the null hypothesis of equal variances at the 5% level ($p = 0.035$). We carry on for the rest of the test but we will certainly not ignore this. We shall pay close attention to the results of the non-parametric test alternative to the one-way ANOVA shortly, in section 9.7.1.

If you go back to the top of Table 9.7 you get the results from the ANOVA. The table for the ANOVA breaks the sum of squares (SS) – explained below – down by source: either between group or within group.

'D.F.' stands for degrees of freedom. The total degrees of freedom is the number of cases minus 1. In this case it is 527 cases – 1 = 526. The between groups degrees of freedom is the number of groups (in this case electoral wards, and there are five of them) minus 1 (i.e. 4 in this case). The within groups degrees of freedom is the difference between the total degrees of freedom and the between groups degrees of freedom; i.e. 526 – 4 = 522.

The next column gives the sum of squares. You should find the following: between SS + within SS = total SS (259970.7134 +

Table 9.7

One way ANOVA for General Health scores by locality

Reported LLI

ONE WAY

Variable GH General Health
By Variable LOCALITY

Analysis of Variance

Source	D.F.	Sum of Squares	Mean Squares	F Ratio	F Prob.
Between Groups	4	12073.2270	3018.3068	6.0605	0.0001
Within Groups	522	259970.7134	498.0282		
Total	526	272043.9404			

Group	Count	Mean	Standard Deviation	Standard Error	95 Pct Conf Int for Mean
Grp 1	48	52.6719	24.0463	3.4708	45.6895 TO 59.6542
Grp 2	174	49.4583	23.5125	1.7825	45.9401 TO 52.9765
Grp 3	101	42.9043	21.2507	2.1145	38.7091 TO 47.0995
Grp 4	67	35.8706	22.9113	2.7991	30.2821 TO 41.4592
Grp 5	137	45.3212	20.5349	1.7544	41.8517 TO 48.7906
Total	527	45.6920	22.7419	0.9907	43.7458 TO 47.6381

Levene Test for Homogeneity of Variances

Statistic	df1	df2	2-tail Sig
2.5989	4	522	0.035

No LLI

ONE WAY

Variable GH General Health
By Variable LOCALITY

Analysis of Variance

Source	D.F.	Sum of Squares	Mean Squares	F Ratio	F Prob.
Between Groups	4	1344.3567	336.0892	1.0618	0.3747
Within Groups	544	172191.0172	316.5276		
Total	548	173535.3739			

Group	Count	Mean	Standard Deviation	Standard Error	95 Pct Conf Int for Mean
Grp 1	53	77.8491	15.6751	2.1531	73.5285 TO 82.1696
Grp 2	177	75.5960	18.4776	1.3889	72.8551 TO 78.3370
Grp 3	116	72.8305	17.8388	1.6563	69.5497 TO 76.1113
Grp 4	59	72.7288	19.0887	2.4851	67.7543 TO 77.7034
Grp 5	144	75.3108	17.0550	1.4212	72.5014 TO 78.1201
Total	549	74.8462	17.7952	0.7595	73.3544 TO 76.3381

Levene Test for Homogeneity of Variances

Statistic	df1	df2	2-tail Sig
0.6454	4	544	0.630

12073.2270 = 272043.9404). The between groups sum of squares is found by calculating the square of the difference between each group mean and the overall mean and then multiplying by the number of cases (people) in that group (locality). The ensuing results (one for each group) are summed. So, for this example, the between SS is calculated as:

$$48 \times (52.6719 - 45.6920)^2 + 174 \times (49.4583 - 45.6920)^2 +$$
$$101 \times (42.9043 - 45.6920)^2 + 67 \times (35.8706 - 45.6920)^2 +$$
$$137 \times (45.3212 - 45.6920)^2 = 12073.2.$$

This gives us the variability between the groups, i.e. how different the groups are.

The within SS is simply the group (locality) variances multiplied by the number of cases (people) in the group minus 1. Remember that the variance is the square of the standard deviation. Hence, it is calculated as:

$$(47 \times 24.0463^2) + (173 \times 23.5125^2) + (100 \times 21.2507^2) +$$
$$(66 \times 22.9113^2) + (136 \times 20.5349^2) = 259970.7$$

This gives us the total variability within the groups, i.e. how different the people within a locality are from each other

The simplest way to get the total SS is to add the between SS and the within SS. The alternative (and more long-winded) way is to subtract each of the individual values from the overall mean and square and sum these. This is the overall variability.

The figure under 'Mean Squares' is the estimated variance and is obtained by dividing the relevant sum of squares by its degrees of freedom. So, the between groups mean squares is 12073.2270 divided by 4, which equals 3018.3. The F-ratio (or F-statistic) is then simply the ratio of the two mean squares, i.e. 3018.3068 / 498.0282, which equals 6.06.

The F–distribution uses two degrees of freedom, the between SS degrees of freedom and the within SS degrees of freedom. As the degrees of freedom increase, the values of the F-distribution converge to one figure and are very similar when the degrees of freedom pass about 100. The 'degrees of freedom' figure for the F-distribution is calculated from the between groups degrees of freedom (4) and the within groups degrees of freedom (522). Computer output tells us that in fact this value for the F-ratio is equivalent to $p = 0.0001$. This, as you will recognize, is highly significant. There appears to be strong evidence for a relationship between ward of residence and GH score for people reporting an LLI. In contrast, the ward means on the GH score for those who reported no LLI in the bottom half of Table 9.7 give a p-value of 0.3747 so we do not reject the null hypothesis that the ward population means are equal for the non-LLI population.

9.6.2 After the ANOVA has been performed

After finding a statistically significant result, as we have above for the LLI group, you may wish to find out which groups differ. Here we return to the problem of multiple comparisons discussed in the last chapter. In our example, there are five wards and if we performed comparisons on all the possible pairs of wards we would be performing 10 comparisons, greatly increasing our chances of a Type I error.

There are a number of options for what are sometimes called '*post hoc* multiple comparisons'. One is called 'least-significant difference', which is equivalent to just performing multiple *t*-tests; i.e. a *t*-test for each pair of wards, 10 in our case. The more popular method is the Bonferroni method, which is a more conservative method. This adjusts for the number of comparisons to be made. It calculates a new p-value based on the number of comparisons to be made. So, for example, if we had 10 comparisons as in our case, if we obtained a p-value of 0.006 from a *t*-test, the adjusted p-value based on Bonferroni's method would be 0.006 multiplied by 10, or 0.06; hence it would not be significant at the 5% level (where $p = 0.05$) as it is now greater than 0.05. For a paired comparison to be significant at the 5% level, the original (before adjustment) p-value would have to be less than 0.05 divided by 10 or 0.005 (0.005 multiplied by 10 equals 0.05). As you can see, for large numbers of comparisons, this method begins to get extremely conservative, i.e. the original p-value would have to be very small to obtain a significant result. In which case it would be wise just to select the groups you are most interested in comparing and ignore the other comparisons to reduce the number of comparisons made.

The Bonferroni adjustment has been criticized not just for its conservatism but because interpretation of results and their significance depends on how many tests are performed. Perneger (1998), for example, believes a better approach is to simply state what tests have been used and why, and allow the readers to come to their own conclusions.

9.6.3 More complex analyses of variance

We have just about reached the limit of the scope of this text in terms of the different analysis of variance versions. Certainly, we have reached the stage where to perform more complicated analyses, which will be mentioned below, it would be wise to stop to get advice. Detailed description here is likely to confuse. Bear in mind also that these also have assumptions such as homogeneity of variance – another reason for obtaining advice before usage.

We shall briefly mention other test procedures that it is possible to perform with variations of ANOVA.

(a) More than one independent variable

So far, we have considered cases where there is just one independent variable to explain one dependent variable. Earlier, we looked at what effect living in different electoral wards had on General Health scores. Prior to that, we considered the effect of marital status on General Health scores. In both cases, we differentiated between those who reported an LLI and those who reported no LLI, and conducted separate analyses. However, what if the distinction between the scores for those with an LLI and scores for those without an LLI was not so clear-cut? Further, what if there was an added effect on General Health scores of having an LLI and being married (or not) on top of the separate effects of reporting an LLI and marital status on General Health scores? Perhaps there is a relationship between having an LLI or not and marital status. The question is, how can we disentangle all these possibilities to get somewhere near the truth?

Well, we can expand the one-way analysis of variance to include more than one independent variable. Remember, the independent variables need to be categorical (nominal or ordinal) and the dependent variables need to be of interval or ratio measurement level. However, we can also include **covariates** in our analysis. This means that we take into account confounding interval- or ratio-level variables. In our example, age could be considered a covariate as it seems that scores worsen in the older age groups. We run an analysis including covariates in the next chapter.

Here, we shall just give a brief description for the case when we have more than one independent categorical variable. We shall be looking at an analysis of variance with the reporting of an LLI or not and marital status as our independent, categorical variables. We have now expanded marital status back into our original variable where people are separated into four categories; 'Married', 'Separated/divorced', 'Widowed' and 'Single'. Consider Table 9.8.

General Health LLI and marital status					
Source of Variation	Sum of Squares	DF	Mean Square	F	Sig of F
Main Effects					
LLI	110909.368	1	110909.368	270.011	0.000
marital	867.888	3	289.296	0.704	0.550
2-Way Interactions					
LLI marital	2960.244	3	986.748	2.402	0.066
Explained	246299.531	7	35185.647	85.660	0.00
Residual	460871.984	1122	410.759		
Total	707171.514	1129	626.370		

Table 9.8

Analysis of variance for General Health scores by LLI status and marital status

Much of it is similar to the one-way ANOVA table. The **main effects** are the two independent factors taken on their own, removing the effect of the other independent factor(s). Here we are testing firstly the null hypothesis that reporting of LLI or not has no effect on General Health scores, and then the null hypothesis that marital status has no effect on General Health scores. However, we are also looking at the effect of the **interaction** of the two variables. What added effect is there, for example, of reporting an LLI and being married?

The concept of interaction is not always easy to comprehend. Indeed, it is not always included in the analysis if it is reasonably believed there will be no interaction effect. However, to understand it, consider the options for a slimmer. Two options are going on a diet and going on to an exercise regime. Both are likely to lead to some weight loss, but what if the most beneficial effects of the diet were from exercising as well? Somebody who diets and exercises may get the individual effects of both, but may also get an added bonus effect. This is the interaction effect. Dieting will have an effect, exercising will have an effect, but the two taken together will have an effect over and above the sum of the individual effects alone.

The degrees of freedom for the main effects are, again, just the number of categories minus 1. So, for LLI it is 2 minus 1, and for marital status there are four possible categories and so there is 3 degrees of freedom. Note that the categories in both of these variables are mutually exclusive. You cannot be in more than one category in either of the two variables. For example, you cannot be in the married category and single; nor can you report an LLI and not report an LLI. Note further that, where a divorced or widowed person has remarried, it is assumed that they will have checked the 'married' option.

The mean squares are as for the one-way ANOVA, i.e. the sum of squares divided by the degrees of freedom. The F-ratio is calculated by dividing the relevant mean square by the residual mean square and the resulting F-ratio (or statistic) is compared to the tables for the F-distribution on the relevant main effect (or interaction) degrees of freedom and the residual degrees of freedom.

In our example in Table 9.8, we can see that, after taking into account the effect of reporting an LLI, marital status does not make a difference. The interaction effect is not quite significant at the 5% level ($p = 0.066$), but it is worth reporting this figure even though, using the conventional 5% level of significance, it is not statistically significant. We saw earlier that, within the LLI group, being married or not does affect General Health score, which is not the case for the non-LLI group.

We do not have to include all interactions. While for a two-variable analysis there is only one interaction, for three variables there will be three two-way interactions (i.e. three pairs of interactions) and one three-way interaction, totalling four altogether. For four variables, there will be six two-way interactions, four three-way interactions and one four-way interaction, totalling 11 interactions. Obviously, the more complicated the interaction the more difficult it is to interpret. The idea is to judge at which level to start the interaction by using common sense. The method is to investigate higher level interactions first, with the null hypothesis that the individual variables in the interaction affect the dependent variable jointly.

SPSS for Windows has two commands for which it is possible to produce these results. They are the simple factorial ANOVA command and the general factorial ANOVA command. The former probably gives the easiest output for the novice to understand. It allows you to choose one or more independent variables and include covariate(s) (to remove the effect of another interval/ratio measured variable on the dependent variable) if needed. The latter allows more flexibility in the construction of the model (e.g. only specifying inclusion of certain interactions).

(b) Final thoughts on ANOVAs

In section 9.6.1 we explained the extension to the independent sample *t*-test, the one way ANOVA. There is also an extension to the paired samples *t*-test.

We could, for example, extend our before intervention/after intervention GH score example to incorporate a new group, namely GH score 6 months after the intervention. Perhaps we would also want to compare two or more interventions as well. Then we need to use a **repeated measures** ANOVA, which is available in SPSS for Windows.

One final thought concerns the situation where you wish to run more than one ANOVA using different dependent variables. If they are uncorrelated then it is best to run different ANOVAs; however, if the dependent variables are related then it is better to run, for example, the MANOVA command in SPSS for Windows (the M stands for 'multivariate'). This takes into account the relationship between the dependent variables as well as assessing the influence of the categorical independent variables.

9.7 NON-PARAMETRIC ALTERNATIVES TO ANOVA

As in the last few sections of the ANOVA descriptions, we shall only give brief descriptions of a couple of the more common non-parametric alternatives to the ANOVA.

9.7.1 The non-parametric alternative to the one-way ANOVA

The **Kruskal–Wallis** test is the extension of the Mann–Whitney test. It assesses whether the mean rank is the same in each group. This test requires that the data has at least an ordinal measurement. The letter given to the test statistic is *H*. The Kruskal–Wallis test is a test for two or more independent groups with at least ordinal measured data. It is calculated in a similar way to the Mann–Whitney test. Indeed, the Kruskal–Wallis test applied to two groups gives us the same results as for the Mann–Whitney test. As in that test, all the values under investigation are ranked in order without regard as to the group they belong in. If the samples come from identical distributions, then the mean ranks of the groups should be approximately the same. The test statistic, *H*, is calculated based on the average rank for each group and this is compared to the relevant value of the chi-square distribution, which we shall pay more attention to later. The degrees of freedom is calculated as the number of groups minus 1.

As for the one-way ANOVA, we will not know where the differences are if we find a significant difference. We could use Mann–Whitney tests afterwards but this will again lead to the problems of multiple testing described above. We shall look at the results of the Kruskal–Wallis test for the comparison of General Health scores by locality as used in our one-way ANOVA demonstration earlier.

Table 9.9

Kruskal–Wallis test for General Health scores by locality

Reported LLI

Kruskal–Wallis 1-Way ANOVA

GH   General Health
by   LOCALITY

Mean Rank	Cases	
308.22	48	Ward A
287.31	174	Ward B
248.26	101	Ward C
199.94	67	Ward D
261.83	137	Ward E
	527	Total

			Corrected for ties		
Chi-Square	D.F.	Significance	Chi-Square	D.F.	Significance
21.0887	4	0.0003	21.1457	4	0.0003

No LLI

Kruskal–Wallis 1-Way ANOVA

GH   General Health
by   LOCALITY

Mean Rank	Cases	
296.66	53	Ward A
284.82	177	Ward B
255.97	116	Ward C
258.53	59	Ward D
277.03	144	Ward E
	549	Total

			Corrected for ties		
Chi-Square	D.F.	Significance	Chi-Square	D.F.	Significance
3.9968	4	0.4064	4.0181	4	0.4036

Table 9.9 gives us the results for both the LLI and non-LLI groups.

As for the Mann–Whitney test we are given the 'mean rank' for each locality and the number of cases (or sample size) for each locality. The chi-square statistic is given for both the standard version and the correction for ties version. As you can see, there is little difference between the two and this is normally the case. The correction for ties actually increases the value of the test statistic, H, and, hence, reduces the p-value. So if the result is significant when a correction is not made it will be significant when a correction for ties is made.

The degrees of freedom ('D.F.') is simply the number of groups minus 1 (i.e. $5 - 1 = 4$). The p-values (or 'Significance') you can see are similar to that for the one-way ANOVA, confirming that within the non-LLI group there appears little effect on scores by locality but that there is in the LLI group. The non-parametric test for the LLI group agrees with the parametric alternative even though we were slightly concerned about the equality of the variances when performing the parametric version.

9.7.2 The non-parametric test for related groups

The extension of the sign and Wilcoxon–Mann–Whitney tests for when there are more than two groups is called the **Friedman test**. There is also the related Kendall W coefficient of concordance. These can be considered the non-parametric equivalent of the repeated-measures ANOVA. Again these tests are based on ranking the data over all the groups as for the Kruskal–Wallis test then calculating the total ranking for each group. The Friedman H statistic is assessed using the chi-square distribution.

Kendall's W ranges from 0 (no association) up to 1 (total association) and gives a similar result.

9.8 A WORD ABOUT THE TESTS IN THIS CHAPTER

We have taken you through a series of tests, including looking at the effect of the values of the independent variables on the dependent variables and adding more variables to the analysis. You would not, in practice, build up through these tests as we have done to exemplify their use. If you have two groups, and common sense and descriptive analysis suggests that there is no confounding variable and the parametric assumptions seem valid, then you should run with one of the t-tests. You should decide beforehand which analysis is appropriate, not run through them all thinking up new variables to analyse.

If you have any confusion or uncertainty when considering any of these methods for use, you should consult a friendly expert for help and advice. Further reading on the parametric procedures can be found in texts such as Altman, 1991 and Wright, 1997. Specialist non-parametric books include Siegel and Castellan, 1988 and Pett, 1997.

Finally, the ANOVA is strongly related to the regression analyses that we will look at in the next chapter.

10 RELATIONSHIPS BETWEEN VARIABLES

10.1 INTRODUCTION

In the previous chapters we have compared statistics between groups. We have compared the value of an interval/ratio scale variable for one group with that of one or more other groups (nominal or ordinal scale variable). We have compared General Health scores from the Short Form-36 between the limiting long-term illness and non-LLI groups, and examined differences in the scores for people of different marital status. We could also, for example, have compared Physical Functioning scores between groups. However, what if we had wanted to assess the relationship between LLI and marital status, both nominal scale variables; or between General Health and Physical Functioning scores, both interval/ratio scale variables? The relationship between variables measured on the same type of scale is what we shall be considering in the first part of this chapter.

Essentially, we shall divide this chapter into three parts. The first part will examine relationships between categorical data (nominal and ordinal), using the chi-square distribution and measuring association. In the second part of the chapter, we will look at relationships between interval/ratio data. We will look at associations or **correlations** between variables measured on this type of scale.

In the final section we shall extend this idea of correlation by taking a look at **regression analysis**. Here, independent variables are modelled to explain and predict values of the dependent variable. For example, we may wish to predict a person's General Health score by looking at their gender, age and Physical Functioning score. There is a family of different regression modelling methods and one of the steps in selecting the most appropriate technique is to look at the scale of measurement of the dependent and independent variables. We shall look at one particular form, namely linear regression analysis, and leave others for further reading or consultation.

10.2 MEASURES OF ASSOCIATION BETWEEN CATEGORICAL DATA

One important aspect of our research was to examine the use of health care services by people reporting a limiting long-term illness. Do people with LLI consult their general practitioner (GP) more or less often than those without LLI? One starting point in examining this is to compare reporting of an LLI with whether the person had consulted their GP in a certain time period (we studied a period of 3 months). A second question addressed whether gender was a factor in consulting. Do women consult more, less or the same as men? Further, does area of residence have an effect on consultation?

To answer questions like this in which both variables are categorical (LLI/non-LLI, consult/not consult, male/female, locality A/locality

B/locality C/, etc.) we need to use a distribution called the **chi-square distribution.**

The symbol of the chi-square distribution is χ^2, which is the Greek letter 'chi' (pronounced with a hard 'k') and the superscript '2' to show the square. The basic idea of the chi-square tests based on this distribution is that they compare the observed data (symbolized by 'O') with data which is calculated as the 'expected' figures (symbolized by 'E'). The resulting chi-square statistic is compared to figures in the chi-square distribution shown in Appendix B, Table B4 to allow testing of our null hypothesis that there is no relationship between the two variables.

If you remember, in Chapter 5 we started building up frequency tables and cross-tabulations or **contingency tables.** When measuring an association the starting point is to draw up a contingency table. For example, in Table 10.1 we have a contingency table which shows whether people who reported an LLI have visited their general practitioner in the previous 3 months, broken down by sex. We can calculate a *p*-value based on the chi-square distribution.

It is easiest to describe and understand measures of association and the chi-square test by considering the simplest form of contingency table, the 2 × 2 table.

For further reading on chi-square based tests, try Everitt, 1992 or a specialist non-parametric book such as Siegel and Castellan, 1988 and Pett, 1997.

10.2.1 Two by two (2 × 2) tables

We asked those who reported an LLI and those who did not whether they had been to see their general practitioner in the previous 3 months. Of the LLI group, 63% (359 out of 573) who answered the question replied that they had, compared to just 37% (219 out of 586) of the non-LLI group. The large difference in proportions suggests that there is an association between visiting your GP in the previous 3 months and reporting an LLI. Consider Table 10.1, taken from our LLI study.

		Female	Male	Total
Visited GP?	Yes	205	154	359
	No	114	100	214
	Total	319	254	573

Table 10.1

Contingency table of observed values from survey for visiting GP by gender within the LLI group

Table 10.1 looks at the LLI group alone and asks the question whether there is any association between seeing a GP and gender; i.e. are women more or less likely to have visited their GP than men (age did not appear to influence GP consultation within the LLI group).

Our null hypothesis (H_0) is that there is no association between visiting a GP and gender within the LLI group in our study population. Our alternative hypothesis (H_1) is that one gender is more likely than the other to have visited the GP within the LLI group. Notice that in our alternative hypothesis we are not saying which gender visits more often.

In Table 10.1, the columns are the gender and the rows are whether a person has visited a GP or not. Each variable has two possible categories (male/female; yes/no) – hence, a two by two table – therefore, everybody is placed into one of four possible compartments. For example, 205 out of the 319 females visited their GP in the previous 3 months.

We could use the Z-test for proportions described in Chapter 8 to assess whether consultation rate was different in men from women. However, the chi-square test is the more common approach and will yield the same results. The Z-test, however, is easier to use to calculate confidence intervals although some statistical packages will give confidence intervals for the difference in proportions when performing a chi-square test. When we have bigger tables than the 2 × 2 table (that is, more than two categories for at least one of the variables) then we cannot use the Z-test.

The chi-square test is based on the **marginal** totals and compares the proportions in each group, i.e. the proportion of females who visited their GP compared to the proportion of males who visited their GP. The marginal totals are the row and column totals. Hence, the row marginal totals are 359 and 214 and the column marginal totals are 319 and 254. The grand total is 573. We can display this table in terms of totals represented by letters, as in Table 10.2, where N represents the grand total, i.e. $a + b + c + d$;

Table 10.2

Contingency table for visiting GP by gender with letters representing counts

		Female	Male	Total
Visited GP?	Yes	a	b	$a + b$
	No	c	d	$c + d$
	Total	$a + c$	$b + d$	N

The first thing we need to do is to calculate the **expected values** based on the marginal totals. This is simply calculated as:

$$\frac{\text{row total} \times \text{column total}}{\text{grand total}}.$$

Therefore, for cell a, the number of females visiting the GP, the expected value is $(359 \times 319) / 573 = 199.86$. This is the number that would occur if the two variables were independent, i.e. if in the LLI group there was no relationship whatsoever between visiting the GP and gender. The expected number of males visiting the GP based on independence of the two variables is $(359 \times 254) / 573 = 159.14$. Table 10.3 shows the table of expected values and the figure underneath in brackets is the **residual**, i.e. the observed value minus the expected value $(O - E)$. If the null hypothesis is true, the observed figure should be very close to the expected figure and the residual will be consequently very small.

		Female	Male	Total	
Visited GP?	Yes	199.86 (5.14)	159.14 (– 5.14)	359	
	No	119.14 (– 5.14)	94.86 (5.14)	214	
	Total	319	254	573	

Table 10.3

Contingency table of expected values (and residuals) for visiting GP by gender within the LLI group

Notice that the marginal totals and the grand totals are the same as in Table 10.1. This has to be the case. Notice also the pattern for the residuals. This is always the case for 2 × 2 tables but only for 2 × 2 tables. The residuals will help us to explain the association if we find sufficient proof for one. A positive residual indicates that the observed figure was greater than expected (greater by the size of the residual) and a negative residual indicates that the observed residual was less than expected (smaller by the size of the residual).

The chi-square statistic is generally calculated by squaring the residual and dividing by the expected value, and summing the results. Hence it is the sum of:

$$\frac{(\text{observed value} - \text{expected value})^2}{\text{expected value}}$$

In this case we get:

$$\chi^2 = \frac{(205 - 199.86)^2}{199.86} + \frac{(154 - 159.14)^2}{159.14} + \frac{(114 - 119.14)^2}{119.14} + \frac{(100 - 94.86)^2}{94.86} = 0.80.$$

Because of the residual property remarked on earlier, the general formula for the calculation of the chi-square statistic can be simplified for the 2 × 2 table to:

$$\chi^2 = \frac{N(ad - bc)^2}{(a+b)(c+d)(a+c)(b+d)}$$

The denominator is, of course, just the product of the marginal totals. Hence, for our example:

$$\chi^2 = \frac{573((205 \times 100) - (114 \times 154))^2}{(359 \times 214 \times 319 \times 254)} = 0.80.$$

Next, we need to calculate the degrees of freedom. This is calculated as

$$(r - 1) \times (c - 1),$$

where r is the number of rows and c is the number of columns. Hence we have $(2 - 1) \times (2 - 1) = 1$ degree of freedom. This has some intuitive logic about it, since if the marginal totals are to remain the same, we can only vary one figure out of the four cells. If we added 1 to 154, then we would automatically need to reduce 205 and 100 by one to keep 359 and 254 as marginal totals, and then 114 would have to increase by one to keep 214 as a marginal total. Another way of thinking about it, in general, is that if you had three figures that had to add up to a certain number (say 10) you could make two of them any numbers you wished but the third would be fixed on the basis of the other two to make sure the sum of 10 was achieved. So, with three figures, there are 2 degrees of freedom.

Another way of calculating the degrees of freedom in a contingency table is to cover up the last row and the last column (within the table – not the marginals) and count the remaining visible cells in the table.

Now we can compare our χ^2 statistic of 0.80 given 1 degree of freedom with the figure for 1 degree of freedom in Table B4 in Appendix B. As you can see, the figure at the 5% level ($\alpha = 0.05$) is 3.841, comfortably above our figure of 0.80. Hence, we do not reject the null hypothesis. Using a computer program gives us a p-value of 0.37. Interestingly, when the same test was performed on those reporting no LLI, there was a significant association between gender and visiting the GP ($p < 0.001$), with females much more likely to consult.

Some authors suggest the use of a standard correction, described first by Frank Yates in 1934, when we have a 2×2 table. For large sample sizes the difference in the result will be slight. SPSS for Windows gives the result both with and without this continuity correction. The result without a continuity correction is called Pearson, after Karl Pearson, who introduced the chi-square test. The continuity correction gives a more conservative result, increasing the p-value. In our example above, it pushed the p-value up slightly to 0.42. If in doubt, i.e. when you are near the required significance level, it is probably better to take the corrected value.

We shall return to 2×2 tables when we consider small expected values.

10.2.2 Larger tables for two variables

The general formulae and structure for two-variable tables apply when we have more than two rows or columns, except where we stated above that it was a special case for 2×2 tables. We calculate the expected value for each in exactly the same way as for the 2×2 table by multiplying the row total by the column total and dividing by the grand total. As before, the chi-square statistic is calculated by squaring each residual, dividing by the expected value and summing the results.

Turning to the LLI example, let us consider SPSS for Windows output for consultation rates by locality. In Table 10.4 we can see the numbers who reported an LLI and visited their GP in the previous 3 months according to the electoral ward in which they live.

Observed Expected Residual		Ward A	Ward B	Ward C	Ward D	Ward E	Total
Visited GP?	Yes	26	102	79	45	83	335
		29.8	113.6	65.4	40.6	85.7	
		− 3.8	− 11.6	13.6	4.4	− 2.7	
	No	21	77	24	19	52	193
		17.2	65.4	37.6	23.4	49.3	
		3.8	11.6	− 13.6	− 4.4	2.7	
Total		47	179	103	64	135	528

Chi-Square	Value	DF	Significance
Pearson	13.88863	4	0.00766

Minimum Expected Frequency – 17.180

Table 10.4

Contingency table of consultation with GP by electoral ward within the LLI group

This is a 2 × 5 table as it has two rows and five columns. The top number in each cell is the observed value (what SPSS for Windows calls 'Count'). The second number is the expected value based on the marginal totals and the null hypothesis that visiting the GP is independent of ward, i.e. that there is no relationship between the two. The final, bottom, figure is the residual, i.e. observed minus expected.

The chi-square calculation is shown beneath the contingency table giving a chi-square statistic of 13.89, on 4 degrees of freedom (calculated as $(2 – 1) \times (5 – 1)$) and a p-value of 0.00766. Can you see how 4 degrees of freedom is arrived at? Therefore, we reject the null hypothesis at the 1% level ($p < 0.01$)and suggest that there is a connection between visiting the GP and ward of residence among those reporting an LLI based on our sample. Examination of the residuals suggests that people in wards C and D were more likely to consult (having positive residuals: observed value is greater than the expected value). These are actually the two most deprived wards out of the five. We have not examined the types of illness here, but some chronic illnesses may not require regular GP attendance, while other people might be receiving secondary care or might have attended the GP for a reason other than for their LLI.

Instead of producing two analyses, one for gender and one for locality, or instead of breaking the sample down into LLI and non-LLI groups and analysing them separately, it is possible to produce a table and analysis for three variables. This, as you might imagine, starts getting a little complicated. We will leave this for further reading.

10.2.3 Limitations of the chi-square test

Problems can arise with the test when the expected values are small. There is no rigid rule as to what 'small' means and Everitt (1992) discusses the various opinions on the matter. As a very general and arbitrary rule, expected values of less than 5 are usually taken to mean that there may be trouble ahead and that the chi-square test may give 'wrong' answers. Cochran (1954) believes that everything should be

OK provided only a relatively small number of cells have expected values less than 5; and one cell in every five or six is usually taken as allowable. More than this may mean the test is not valid, and **all** cells should have expected frequencies greater than 1. SPSS for Windows tells you the minimum calculated expected frequency and how many (if any) cells have expected values less than 5. If there appear to be too many, then two different solutions can be considered, as follows.

It may be necessary to merge columns or rows if it makes sense to do so, in order to increase the values in the cells giving problems. For example, we could merge people who are single, divorced/separated and widowed into one non-married category. Remember, however, that this will change your null hypothesis. We would now be comparing the second variable with whether it was associated with being married or not, rather than with different categories of marital status.

Often age is given as an age grouping (e.g. 35–44) and there may be small numbers in the highest age groups. So we might decide to combine the highest age groups into one group of, say, 75 years and over. Remember, though, that we lose information by merging categories, as we do by categorizing continuous or discrete data. However, it may be the only option.

An alternative solution for 2 × 2 tables is called **Fisher's exact test**, developed by Sir Ronald Fisher, whom we have already met. Fisher's test calculates the probability of the smallest cell count occurring or a smaller one, if, in fact, the null hypothesis of no association is true.

Study Table 10.5, which is taken from our hospital satisfaction survey.

Table 10.5

Contingency table of complaints following hospital visit by sex

Observed Expected Residual		Female	Male	Total
Complained? Yes		5	2	7
		3.5	3.5	
		1.5	− 1.5	
	No	20	23	43
		21.5	21.5	
		− 1.5	1.5	
Total		25	25	50

Chi-Square	Value	DF	Significance
Pearson	1.49502	1	0.22144
Fisher's Exact Test:			
One-Tail			0.20871

Minimum Expected Frequency – 3.500
Cells with Expected Frequency < 5 – 2 OF   4 (50.0%)

It examines whether there is more or less dissatisfaction among women compared with men. You can see that two of the four cells (both the complaints 'yes' cells) have expected values less than 5 (3.5, to be exact).

The results from Fisher's exact test are given (we shall leave it to further reading for details of calculation). This is, unlike the chi-square test, a one-tailed test (χ^2 is a two-tailed test). In this case, while the null hypothesis is the same (dissatisfaction is independent of gender) the alternative hypothesis for the exact test is that proportionally more females than males complained. On the basis of this data, we cannot say that there is an association between dissatisfaction and gender, as the p-value is greater than 0.05.

10.2.4 Final thoughts on the chi-square test

The chi-square is one of those things that starts from a very simple premise but can build up to be quite complicated. We have only touched upon the many applications of the chi-square test. For example, we have not covered the χ^2 for trend test for ordinal data (see, for example, Altman, 1991). This is for the situation when one of the variables is ordered, since it takes that order into account. Neither have we looked at the state of affairs when the data is matched, such as comparing before and after an intervention, and the use of **McNemar's test**.

Finally, remember association does not mean causation. We shall return to this later.

And so to **correlation**.

10.3 RELATIONSHIPS BETWEEN TWO INTERVAL/RATIO-MEASURED VARIABLES

A clinician wanders up to us late one afternoon and says to us that it is very interesting to know the various effects that marital status and ward of residence have on SF-36 scale scores, but he is also interested in knowing whether people who score badly on the physical-type scales also score badly on the mental-type scales of the SF-36. This now leads us into a different type of analysis. We no longer have two or three defined groups between which to compare a particular variable. Now we have variables all of the interval/ratio type and we wish to discover whether any relationships exist between them.

Remember the scatterplot that we described in Chapter 5, suitable for data measured on an interval or ratio scale? Well, such a plot graphically displays the relationship between two interval/ratio variables, one measured on the y (vertical)-axis and one measured on the x (horizontal)-axis.

Consider the six parts of Figure 10.1, all showing hypothetical plots with different variables measured against each other.

Take each one in turn and, before carrying on reading, consider what you feel is the relationship between the two variables in each plot.

You should see clear signs of a relationship in at least five of them. Figures 10.1(a) and 10.1(b) are perfectly straight lines and this indicates **perfect correlation**. Figure 10.1(a) is called perfect positive correlation since an increase in the value of one variable is met by an equivalent increase in the other variable. In Figure 10.1(b) we have a perfect negative correlation as an increase in the value of one variable

Figure 10.1

Scatterplots representing different size associations. (a) $r = +1$, perfect positive correlation. (b) $r = -1$, perfect negative correlation. (c) $r = 0.85$, strong positive correlation. (d) $r = -0.55$, negative correlation. (e) $r = 0.06$, no correlation. (f) $r = 0$, strong non-linear relationship.

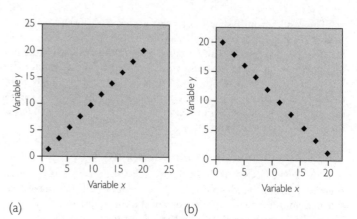

(a)   (b)

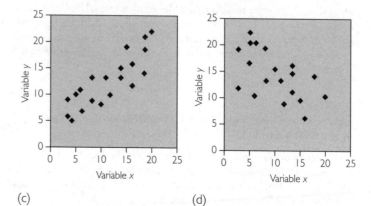

(c)   (d)

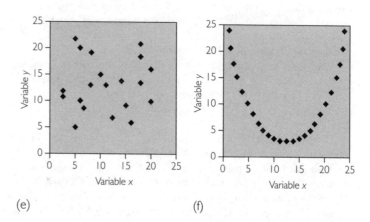

(e)   (f)

is met by an equivalent decrease in the other variable. Figure 10.1(c) also illustrates a positive correlation, while Figure 10.1(d) concerns negative correlation, but neither is as 'tidy' as their neighbours in Figures 10.1(a) and 10.1(b) respectively. However, there does appear to be an approximate straight line (or **linear**) relationship. Height and weight, for example, tend to be quite strongly positively correlated. A positive correlation in general means that a high value on one variable tends to be matched by a high value on the other, and a low value on one variable tends to be matched with a low value on the other. A negative correlation in general means that a high value of one variable tends to be matched by a low value on the other variable and vice versa. Figure 10.1(e) is much more of a haphazard pattern and there is no real discernible correlation between the two variables. Figure 10.1(f) has an unusual relationship, but there does appear to be a relationship, to which we shall come back shortly

Those types of analysis, as with the various t-tests and the Wilcoxon, sign and Mann–Whitney tests, are forms of **bivariate analysis**, i.e. we are studying two variables. We do not have to rely only on eyeballing a scatterplot to assess the strength of the association between two variables, as there are two commonly used statistics which summarize the association in one figure, one based on parametric assumptions and one based on non-parametric assumptions. We shall consider the parametric version first.

10.3.1 Pearson's product moment correlation coefficient

The most common **correlation coefficient** is that devised by Karl Pearson and is denoted by the letter r. This is an estimate (based on sample data) of the population correlation coefficient, ρ (rho). It is a measure of association based on measuring the linear (straight-line) relationship between two variables. It is the parametric version for use when the variables have a normal distribution. Pearson's r requires that both variables are measured on an interval/ratio scale. It is not appropriate when there is a different type of relationship, i.e. non-linear. (However, all is not lost, since it may be reasonable to transform the data to a more linear pattern. A transformation is carried out by performing a mathematical operation on each value of a variable, such as taking the natural log of each value. This should be done in consultation with someone who has specialist knowledge.)

The value of r ranges from -1 to $+1$. The closer the figure gets to either -1 or $+1$, the more 'perfect' the relationship. A value for r of 1 indicates a perfectly positive correlation, as shown in the scatterplot in Figure 10.1(a). That is, all the points fall on a straight line from bottom-left to top-right. A value for r of -1 indicates a perfectly negative correlation, as shown in the scatterplot in Figure 10.1(b), i.e. all the points fall on a straight line from top left to bottom right. For both values, $r = 1$ and $r = -1$, we can predict perfectly the value of one variable from the other. These, as you might expect, are rare situations and the scenarios presented in Figure 10.1(c)–(e) are more common. Figures 10.1(c) and 10.1(d) have r values of 0.85 and -0.55 respectively, showing some relationships – but not perfect ones. There is very little relationship between the variables in Figure 10.1(e), indicated by the *r* value of 0.06. One thing to point out is that *r* is unitless. It does not matter if the variables are measured on different scales (e.g. height in centimetres and weight in grams).

Now look at Figure 10.1(f). The *r* value is zero, which suggests that there is no relationship. But this is not actually right. It suggests that there is no **linear** relationship, but our visual perusal of the scatterplot suggests a non-linear relationship. The message is not to get into the habit of relying solely on *r* values; always plot the points and look for non-linear as well as linear relationships.

It is possible to produce a correlation matrix that shows the bivariate relationships between a number of different variables, when the variables are all measured on an interval/ratio scale. Table 10.6 shows the correlation between the scale scores on the SF-36.

Table 10.6

Pearson's correlation coefficient matrix for scales of the SF-36

	Phys. Funct.	Role – Phys.	Role – Emot.	Bodily Pain	Gen. Health	Vitality	Social Funct.	Mental Health
Phys. Funct.	1.00							
Role – Phys.	0.73	1.00						
Role – Emot.	0.45	0.58	1.00					
Bodily pain	0.66	0.70	0.43	1.00				
Gen. Health	0.70	0.66	0.46	0.66	1.00			
Vitality	0.61	0.60	0.54	0.59	0.72	1.00		
Social Funct.	0.65	0.66	0.62	0.61	0.65	0.70	1.00	
Mental Health	0.34	0.35	0.56	0.36	0.51	0.63	0.56	1.00

It is a triangular matrix, as the other half of the matrix is symmetrical to the first (it does not matter which variable is taken as the first variable, or the *y*-variable). Obviously, a variable correlated with itself will have an *r* value of 1. The matrix in Table 10.6 shows the higher correlations between the physical scales (e.g. Physical Functioning and Role Limitations – Physical has a value of *r* of 0.73) than between the physical and mental scales (e.g. Physical Functioning and Mental Health has a value of *r* of 0.34). Indeed, Mental Health seems to have the weakest linear association with the other scales. Also notice, as might be expected, that all the correlations are positive (i.e. if you score highly on one scale, you also tend to score highly on the other scales).

It is possible to assess the evidence for the relationship between two variables in a population by a hypothesis test. The null hypothesis is that there is no association (i.e. that ρ, the population correlation coefficient, equals 0). We therefore assess the strength of evidence against this null hypothesis being true, on the basis of our sample data. However, for large sample sizes, even apparently small correlations can give statistically significant results, implying that there is some linear association. For example, with a sample size of 100, a value for *r* of 0.2 will be significant (i.e. rejecting the null hypothesis) at the 5% level and a value of 0.3 will be significant at the 1% level. This can mean that small correlations are regarded as important when all we should be saying is that there probably is some association but it is a weak one.

There is also the problem of multiple testing when some of the tests might be significant by chance because of the number of tests we are performing. For example, we only have eight SF-36 scales in Table 10.6 but this equates to 28 pairings and, hence, 28 tests. Often, only the r value is given, rather than the additional hypothesis test. There is no clear rule about which value of r denotes a strong relationship. It is also possible to calculate a confidence interval for r.

The calculation of Pearson's r is tedious to perform by hand and we will assume that you will use your friendly statistical computer software or spreadsheet to calculate it for you.

10.3.2 The non-parametric alternative to Pearson's r

The alternative to Pearson's r, which is often seen in articles and papers in journals, is **Spearman's rank-order correlation coefficient**, denoted by r_s. This has fewer assumptions than Pearson's r and is suitable for use when both variables are measured on at least an ordinal scale. The advantage of Spearman's coefficient is that the two variables do not have to be linearly related, just that an increase in one variable will see an increase or decrease in the other (known as a monotonic relationship). As its name suggests, and in common with most other non-parametric techniques, it is based on ranking each case according to each of the two variables. Like Pearson's r, the value of r_s ranges from -1 to $+1$. Hypothesis tests can again be made, based on the null hypothesis that there is no association between the two variables. If parametric assumptions are justified and the variables are linearly related, then Spearman's r_s is considered inferior to Pearson's r as it uses less of the data (being based on the ranks of the data rather than the data itself). Pearson's r, as we shall see shortly, is also used in linear regression analysis.

If parametric assumptions hold, the two alternatives should be similar. One way to produce a rough test of these assumptions is to calculate both the Pearson and Spearman's correlation coefficients. If they are similar, then there is good reason to believe that the variables are normally distributed. Spearman's rank-order correlation coefficient is actually just Pearson's correlation coefficient calculated on the ranks of the data rather than the actual data itself.

Table 10.7 shows the correlation matrix for the SF-36 scale scores using Spearman's correlation coefficient. The results are very similar to Pearson's correlation coefficient and so we can be confident in using Pearson's r.

Another non-parametric correlation procedure, less commonly used than Pearson's or Spearman's, is Kendall's rank-order correlation coefficient, tau τ. This is similar to Spearman's in that the variables have to be measured on at least ordinal scale and it is based on the rankings of the variables. Again, it ranges from -1 to $+1$ and the interpretation of the value of tau is the same as for Pearson's r. For more details on Kendall's tau, see Petit, 1997 or Siegel and Castellan, 1988.

Table 10.7

Spearman's correlation coefficient matrix for scales of the SF-36

	Phys. Funct.	Role – Phys.	Role – Emot.	Bodily Pain	Gen. Health	Vitality	Social Funct.	Mental Health
Phys. Funct.	1.00							
Role – Phys.	0.72	1.00						
Role – Emot.	0.41	0.56	1.00					
Bodily Pain	0.67	0.69	0.41	1.00				
Gen. Health	0.69	0.64	0.45	0.64	1.00			
Vitality	0.61	0.62	0.54	0.59	0.73	1.00		
Social Funct.	0.60	0.68	0.62	0.61	0.65	0.68	1.00	
Mental Health	0.34	0.36	0.54	0.37	0.52	0.63	0.55	1.00

10.3.3 Partial correlation

One disadvantage of bivariate (two-variable) correlation is that we do not know, if we find a relationship between two variables, whether this is because there is a genuinely strong relationship between them or because they are both strongly related to a third variable. For example, Physical Functioning and Role Limitations due to Physical Problems may be highly correlated simply because they are both related to age, with older age equating to worse scale scores (age here would be a confounder of the apparent relationship between physical functioning and role limitations – the 'alternative explanation'). Perhaps the Mental Health scale is not highly correlated with age, hence its smaller association with other scales.

Both Pearson's r and Kendall's tau can be adapted to allow for partial correlation, i.e. removing the effects of a suspected third variable related to both the other two. In effect, we are 'controlling' for the third variable.

Table 10.8 repeats the analysis of Table 10.6 using Pearson's r but removes the effect of age on the two variables. There is a very slight fall in the correlation coefficients.

Table 10.8

Pearson's correlation coefficient matrix for scales of the SF-36 adjusted for age

	Phys. Funct.	Role – Phys.	Role – Emot.	Bodily Pain	Gen. Health	Vitality	Social Funct.	Mental Health
Phys. Funct.	1.00							
Role – Phys.	0.68	1.00						
Role – Emot.	0.43	0.57	1.00					
Bodily Pain	0.65	0.68	0.42	1.00				
Gen. Health	0.67	0.63	0.44	0.64	1.00			
Vitality	0.59	0.58	0.53	0.57	0.71	1.00		
Social Funct.	0.63	0.63	0.61	0.59	0.62	0.67	1.00	
Mental Health	0.35	0.36	0.57	0.38	0.51	0.64	0.57	1.00

Snedecor and Cochran (1980) give a nice example of the effects of a third variable on two correlated variables. They report a study that found statistically significant correlations from a study of 142 women between age and blood pressure, age and cholesterol concentration in the blood and blood pressure and cholesterol concentration in the blood. This last correlation was examined more closely. Recognizing the effect of age on both blood pressure and cholesterol concentration in the blood, it was hypothesized that blood pressure and cholesterol concentration in the blood might be related only because of their common association with age. The effects of age were then removed by partial correlation and the correlation between blood pressure and cholesterol concentration in the blood fell to 0.1 and was no longer statistically significant.

10.3.4 Some thoughts on correlation

It must be remembered that association does not mean cause. All we find in correlation is association; we cannot prove causation. If we found a positive relationship between alcohol consumption and weight, this might mean that drinking causes you to put on more weight, or that being heavier makes you drink more, or that there is a hidden confounder to explain the observation.

We also need to be aware about spurious associations. Consider whether the association actually makes sense. For example, we may find that there is a negative correlation between sales of fridge-freezers and infant mortality, i.e. while sales of fridge-freezers have risen, infant mortality has fallen. To say that there is an association between the two is far too simplistic.

When we see a high correlation, either positive or negative, we need to use common sense and judge whether it is actually plausible. Further, we may be interested in searching the literature to see whether other studies have found similar correlations. We should always consider whether there is a third variable strongly related to both of the other two that may be causing this high correlation.

Finally, you may have noticed that we did not differentiate between the LLI and non-LLI groups in our correlation example of the SF-36 scales scores. In this case we are looking at the overall scores. This is actually hiding some interesting information which only comes out when you analyse the two groups separately. For example, there is actually a stronger association between General Health score and Physical Functioning score in the LLI group ($r = 0.61$) than in the non-LLI group ($r = 0.40$). More problems would have been created if the relationship had been different in the two groups, one positively correlated and one negatively correlated, for example. Then we would have obtained a totally misleading value for r. Simple scatterplots of any groupings (e.g. one scatterplot of General Health against Physical Functioning for the LLI group and one for the non-LLI group) should help reveal anything untoward.

10.4 REGRESSION ANALYSIS

Now that we have discovered apparently strong relationships between different SF-36 scale scores, we may be interested in knowing if we can predict or estimate a scale score, say General Health (GH), on the basis of the values of the other scale scores and perhaps the reporting of LLI or not, gender and age also being used to predict the GH score. This leads us to one of the most popular forms of statistical analysis, regression analysis. This is fairly easy to perform with a statistical package but very difficult to perform correctly, and there are a number of assumptions, which are often ignored and can lead to improper conclusions resulting from the analysis.

In this section we look at linear regression analysis, which assumes a linear (straight line) relationship between a dependent variable and one or more independent variables. The dependent variable must be measured on an interval/ratio scale and the independent variables on an interval/ratio scale or a dichotomous (e.g. Yes/No, Male/Female) scale. We want to see how well we can predict the value of the dependent variable (e.g. GH scale score) working from the values of the independent variables (e.g. PF scale score, age, reporting of LLI or not, or gender).

In the medical world we are unlikely to come across a situation where the true relationship is perfectly linear, but we hope to be able to approximate a linear relationship by using a linear model.

What follows does not address all the complexities of simple linear regression analysis and multiple regression analysis, and we suggest that readers who wish to use these techniques seek advice and study the further reading in addition.

10.4.1 One independent variable

If you look back at Figure 10.1(a) and (b) we could perfectly predict the value of the y variable if we knew the value of the x variable (and vice versa). This is because the points fall on a perfectly straight line (we have perfect correlation, a linear relationship). However, this is unrealistic in normal, everyday situations and we are more likely to come across the plots in Figure 10.1(c)–(f). In Figures 10.1(c) and (d) we could estimate what the value of y is if we knew the value of x (and vice versa) but we could not be sure we were correct. Just by eyeballing the scatterplots we could draw a straight line through the plots that seems to best represent the data, as we have done in Figure 10.2. We could then use this line to estimate a value for y based on our value for x by drawing a line up from the value of x on the x-axis to the line and then across to the y-axis to get the predicted value of y.

However, you can see that we would get some errors in our predicted values: the dots are not all on our fitted line. You may also have drawn a slightly different line through the data. Simple linear regression analysis, therefore, considers these errors and tries to draw the 'line of best fit' or, in other words, to calculate the best model for the sample data, the model that best estimates the values of the dependent variable. Linear regression analysis derives a formula for the 'line of best fit'.

It is customary to predict variable y based on variable x. If you look at our 'best guess' line in Figure 10.2, you will see that the line, if extended, would not cross the axis at the origin (i.e. where both x and y equal zero and the x-axis and y-axis meet). Therefore, there is a value of y (known as a constant) where the line crosses the y-axis (known as the intercept) where $x = 0$. Let us call that constant α. The slope of the line is also important in our prediction of the value of y; let us therefore call the slope of the line β. Finally, because it is not a perfect relationship, we know that we are likely to make some error (hopefully small) in our prediction of y from x. This error, the difference between the actual and predicted value, is known more correctly as a **residual** and is denoted by e.

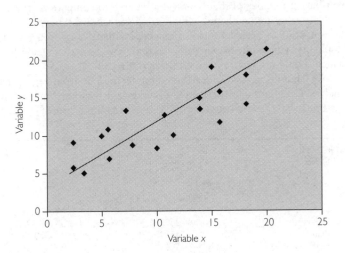

Figure 10.2

Visually estimated line of 'best fit'.

We wish to use our sample data to estimate the values of α and β. As we used the sample data to estimate the population mean and variance, so we are using the sample data to calculate estimates of the population values of α and β, these estimates being denoted by a and b respectively.

Linear regression analysis uses a technique called least squares to calculate these estimates of α and β. We will not go into the precise calculation in regression analysis, but interested readers can go to texts such as Altman, 1991 or Wright, 1997 or a specialized book on regression analysis.

Take as an example the scatterplot of Physical Functioning (PF) score against General Health (GH) score in Figure 5.7. The first thing to do when performing regression analysis is to simply plot the data. Draw a scatterplot of the two variables and assess whether you can see any linear relationship. In Figure 5.7 we can see that there appears to be some kind of linear relationship between the two scale scores but obviously not a strong one. The Pearson correlation coefficient for these two variables is 0.70, which suggests a reasonable positive correlation. When drawing this initial scatterplot, we also need to consider whether there are any outliers or unusual values. These may have a large impact on the resulting statistic and they will need to be checked to see whether they are mistakes in measurement or data recording or whether they are true outliers. For example, if we came across someone with a height of 259 cm we would be confident that it was an error; perhaps a '2' was typed by mistake instead of a '1'. If we came across a height of 195 cm we could not be so sure it was a mistake rather than an outlier. In both situations we would need to go back to the raw data to check the real value. If they are true outliers, then a decision must be made as to whether to remove them from the analysis. If they are errors we should correct them before the regression is performed. Outliers may pull the true regression line towards their values and so, if you have a number of them, it would be wise to compare regression analyses calculated with and without outliers included. However, you do not want to keep removing supposed 'outliers' until you get the result that you want. In our case, we only have one obvious outlier, which should not have a great effect on our results.

We should now consider the computer output from regression analysis given in Table 10.9, and look under the heading 'Variables in the Equation' (we shall consider the rest of the output shortly).

Table 10.9

Regression analysis of General Health with Physical Functioning as the independent variable

Multiple R	0.70165
R Square	0.49231
Adjusted R Square	0.49186
Standard Error	17.90517

Analysis of Variance

	DF	Sum of Squares	Mean Square
Regression	1	350988.95853	350988.95853
Residual	1129	361951.98993	320.59521

F = 1094.80413   Signif F = 0.0000

Variables in the Equation

Variable	B	SE B	95%	Confdnce Intrvl B	Beta
PF	0.557653	0.016854	0.524585	0.590721	0.701649
(Constant)	22.131321	1.276610	19.626526	24.636116	

Variable	Tolerance	VIF	T	Sig T
PF	1.000000	1.000	33.088	0.0000
(Constant)			17.336	0.0000

We have the entered variables and their coefficients; their values for a and b (given under B in the computer output). In Table 10.9 we can see that for one independent variable (PF score) the model is GH = 22.1313 + 0.5577PF; a (the constant) = 22.1313, b (the slope) = 0.5577. As for population means and proportions, it is possible to calculate 95% confidence intervals for these values (go back to Chapter 8 if you need to refresh your memory about confidence intervals). This confidence interval tells us the range we could confidently expect the population variables, α and β, which we are estimating by a and b, to fall in.

More generally, the estimated General Health score is 22.1313 + (0.5577 × Physical Functioning score). Therefore, the model gives us an estimate of 22.1313 for α and 0.5577 for β. Each increase of 1 in PF score, therefore, increases the estimated GH score by 0.5577. So, selecting randomly from our sample, let us say we select Mrs K who has a PF score of 80. What would we predict her GH score to be? Well, we just substitute it into our model and we get an estimated GH score of = 22.1313 + (0.5577 × 80) = 66.75. Her actual score was 60 so we have a residual of just under 7, not a bad prediction on this occasion for this person.

10.4.2 More than one independent variable (multiple regression)

We can, of course, use more than one independent variable to estimate or predict the value of our dependent variable. Indeed, we would expect that we might get a better estimate by using more than one independent variable since there are few situations where using just one independent variable will give a good predictive model.

This type of linear regression analysis is called **multiple regression analysis**. Here, each variable gets its own estimate, denoted by b, associated with it.

One assumption of this type of model is that each of the independent variables has a linear relationship with the dependent variable. So we should plot each independent variable against the dependent variable to assess whether there appears to be a straight line relationship. Also, we should plot the independent variables against each other and seek relationships between them. If there is a lot of correlation between them, then we may run into problems.

Let us add more variables in to our model to predict GH. If we let Physical Functioning (PF) represent the physical side of general health, then let us use the Mental Health (MH) scale to represent the mental aspect of general health. These two scales have been found to be the best indicators of physical and mental health, respectively (Ware *et al.*, 1993). We shall also add in age and two dichotomous variables: reporting of a limiting long-term illness or not (where 0 represents no LLI and 1 represents reported LLI) and sex (where 0 represents female and 1 represents male). Notice, when using a dichotomous variable, that we use 0 and 1 (absence or presence of a particular characteristic). If we used 1 and 2, the regression analysis would take this to be on an interval/ratio scale and, for example, those with an LLI would be regarded as twice those without an LLI if reporting of LLI was given a value of 2 and reporting no LLI was given a value of 1. We could include categorical variables with more than two categories by using what are known as **dummy** variables. For example, if you consider locality where we have five electoral wards, we could have a variable 'wardA' where a '1' is allocated to a person if they live in ward A and '0', otherwise. Then, a variable 'wardB' where a '1' is allocated to a person if they live in ward B and '0', otherwise. Similarly for wardC and wardD. If someone lived in ward E, they would score '0' on all the four variables wardA to wardD; hence we do not need a separate variable for ward E.

Multiple regression works by estimating the effect of one independent variable on the dependent variable after eliminating the effects of the other independent variables. Hence, for example, Physical Functioning score will have its effect on General Health score assessed after removing the effects on the General Health score of Mental Health score, age, gender and reporting of an LLI or not.

Table 10.10

Regression analysis of General Health by Physical Functioning, Mental Health, age, sex and LLI

Multiple R	0.79069	
R Square	0.62519	
Adjusted R Square	0.62351	
Standard Error	15.42056	

Analysis of Variance

	DF	Sum of Squares	Mean Square
Regression	5	442658.24075	88531.64815
Residual	1116	265377.87656	237.79380
F = 372.30428	Signif F = 0.0000		

Variables in the Equation

Variable	B	SE B	95% Confdnce Intrvl B		Beta
LLI	− 11.743571	1.145790	− 13.991717	− 9.495425	− 0.233725
AGE	0.008741	0.034244	− 0.058449	0.075931	0.005221
SEX	− 4.580686	0.934255	− 6.413780	− 2.747591	− 0.090867
MH	0.410132	0.026204	0.358716	0.461547	0.308260
PF	0.379905	0.020123	0.340423	0.419388	0.474998
(Constant)	12.189270	3.241605	5.828943	18.549598	

Variable	Tolerance	VIF	T	Sig T
LTILL	0.645840	1.548	− 10.249	0.0000
AGE	0.802724	1.246	0.255	0.7986
SEX	0.977837	1.023	− 4.903	0.0000
MH	0.865784	1.155	15.651	0.0000
PF	0.530572	1.885	18.880	0.0000
(Constant)			3.760	0.0002

The equation we are left with after the regression analysis is shown under 'Variables in the Equation':

Estimated GH = 12.1893 + 0.3799PF + 0.4101MH + 0.0087age − 11.7436LLI − 4.5807sex.

The constant (*a*) is 12.1893, and each of the other variables has its particular slope (*b*), having taken account of the influence of the other variables in the equation.

Notice the negative coefficients for LLI and sex, which suggest that reporting an LLI or being a male worsens your GH score, since it reduces the predicted GH score. High PF score or a high MH score or being older seem to improve the score. However, this seems to go against what we know about the relationship between age and SF-36 scores found earlier. Looking at the model we can see that each extra year increases the predicted GH score by only 0.0087 so, on this basis, an 80-year-old with the same values for the other variables in the equation as a 30-year-old will score only (50 × 0.0087) or 0.435 higher on GH, predicted by our model. Age, therefore, does not seem to add to our model after the effects of the other variables are taken into account. This is probably because it is highly related to LLI and other SF-36 scales.

Remember Mrs K? Well, she is a 40-year-old female (female value is '0') who reported LLI (value '1') and has a MH score of 60. Let us substitute these into the above equation.

Predicted GH = 12.1893 + 0.3799(80) + 0.4101(60) + 0.0087(40) − 11.7436(1) − 4.5807(0) = 55.79. Our residual has dropped to just over 4 (remember she actually scored 60 on GH). A slight improvement.

This equation means that reporting an LLI (inserting a '1' in the equation) reduces predicted GH score by 11.7436, being a male decreases it by 4.5807, while, for example, every extra score of 1 on PF increases the GH score by 0.3799.

We also have a value for a measure denoted by 'beta' in Table 10.10. This is a standardization technique that allows you to compare the different effects of variables when the coefficients for the variables are measured in different units (e.g. height in centimetres and weight in grams). So, in Table 10.10 we can see that PF has the highest value for beta, which indicates that it has the biggest influence on the model, and, as we suspected, age has the least effect, with sex also having little effect.

10.4.3 Selecting a model

We shall combine ideas of how to select a model with looking at some of the output from a regression analysis. Table 10.9 gives the output when we regress only PF on GH. Table 10.10 gives the output when we use variables PF, MH, age, sex and LLI to predict General Health score. Currently, when we have more than one independent variable, as in Table 10.10, we are simply entering all the variables. However, there are methods to assess the fit of different models based on different selections of independent variables.

The first part of the output in Tables 10.9 and 10.10 considers the fit of the model. This is based on the R or r statistic we encountered earlier. When we have just the one independent variable, the figure to look at is the 'R Square' or R^2, which is simply Pearson's correlation coefficient between the dependent and independent variable, multiplied by itself. This figure indicates how much of the variation within the dependent variable (in our case, General Health score) is accounted for by the independent variable. For example, with PF it means how much PF scores explain the differing GH scores of the subjects. It is sometimes known as the **coefficient of determination**. The closer to 1 it is, the better the fit of the model. As it is a square of R it will always be positive between 0 and 1. In Table 10.9 it is 0.49 and so we can say that the independent variable accounts for 49% of the variation in the dependent variable. This is not a brilliant fit but does indicate some linear relationship between the two variables. The value we would be happy with depends on the situation and how tight a fit we are looking for. Notice that the value for R is the same as the correlation coefficient between GH and PF we considered earlier.

The analysis of variance test (shown below the R^2) tests the null hypothesis that the R^2 figure for the **population** model is equal to zero (i.e. that there is no linear relationship between the variables – there may be a non-linear relationship, though). We have a highly significant result, 'Signif = 0.0000' (the p-value), so we can assume that the population R^2 is not zero.

When we start adding variables to our model, as in Table 10.10, the figure for R^2 will increase even if the new variable adds nothing to our model. The more independent variables there are, the higher R^2 will be. Therefore, the value of R^2 will be artificially high. To adjust for this, a new variable called the adjusted R^2 can be calculated and should be the one used for multiple independent variables. In Table 10.10 this value is 0.62, meaning that the fit of the model has now improved and explains 62% of the variation in the dependent variable.

One way to select the model is simply to run different regression analyses based on different subsets of the independent variables, compare the adjusted R^2 values and use common sense to interpret them, picking the best model for your purposes.

At the bottom of Tables 10.9 and 10.10 there are t-tests for the null hypothesis that the population coefficient (β) for the respective variable is zero. This is a test of whether there is any relationship between that variable and the dependent variable and whether adding it explains any extra variability. The null hypothesis is that there is no relationship. Does the inclusion of the variable improve the model or can it be left out of the model without harming the model? It compares the model that includes this variable to the one where this variable (and only this variable) is removed. As you can see from Table 10.10, it appears that age has little or no impact on the model, having a p-value of 0.7986, which is comfortably above the conventional 0.05 used as the upper limit for statistical significance. We cannot reject the null hypothesis that its β coefficient is zero. Therefore, we can quite safely drop it from the model. You may see an F-statistic rather than a t-statistic used (or both) for the testing of each individual independent variable in some packages; the F-statistic, in this case, is simply the square of the t-statistic.

The methods of selection used in statistical packages tend to be based on these t-tests, which assess the significance of a variable; i.e. test the null hypothesis that its population coefficient, β, is zero. A rather arbitrary p-value is chosen as the boundary from beneath which variables are chosen. Often, this is the traditional 0.05. We shall use this value in our example.

There are a number of methods for carrying out this selection and testing of each set of variables, but three are commonly used in the popular statistical computer packages; forward regression, backward regression and stepwise regression. You select only the variables you want to be considered and then the computer software will select from them the variables giving the best model.

In forward regression, we start with no variables in the model. The variable with the strongest association with the dependent variable will be selected by the computer, i.e. the variable with the smallest p-value, provided it is less than 0.05 (or whatever value we have selected) on the t-test. We recalculate the model including this variable and then the next most associated independent variable is selected. This will explain the greatest amount of the remaining variability. We continue adding variables until none has a p-value smaller than our set limit (e.g. 0.05).

In backward regression, we do the opposite. We start off with all the variables in the model and remove the one that accounts for the least variability; in other words, it has the least association with the dependent variable (i.e. has the largest p-value). Again we continue until, this time, no variable has an associated p-value above our limit (perhaps 5% or 0.05 again). Often, backward and forward regression will yield the same model, but it need not necessarily be the case.

The final method is called stepwise regression. It is a mixture of forward and backward regression. Here, we start with no variables in the model and add variables as with forward regression. However, after each stage, when a variable is entered, we check to see that none of the variables currently in the model should now be removed, as in backward regression. We stop when no more variables can be added or removed, working from our limit for the p-value. Note that we can set different values for p for entry and removal.

Table 10.11 shows the final model from a stepwise regression and the order in which variables were added. As we suspected before, we do not need age in the model. As well as being associated with GH, it is strongly associated with reporting of an LLI and the PF score, and, after these two variables have been added, its partial effect is small.

The new model, therefore, is GH = 12.7588 + 0.3780PF + 0.4110MH − 11.7372LLI − 4.5851sex, which gives Mrs K a predicted GH score of 55.92 − very little different from the situation when age was included in the model.

The criticism levelled at the above computer-based approaches is that they are very much hands-off approaches. You sit back and wait for the computer to select a model for you, although you may have different criteria from the computer for what makes the best model. It also means that you are having less say in how your data is analysed: you do not select the variables to be included in the final model, the computer does. For example, the computer may select one variable rather than another because there is a very slightly better association with the dependent variable. However, the non-selected variable may be more relevant for your situation than the one selected. You have to be very careful in how you interpret the final model selected for you and in the variables you choose for the original set of independent variables from which the model is selected.

Table 10.11	**Step**	**Mult R**	**R sq.**	**F (Eqn)**	**Sig. F**	**Variable**	**BetaIn**
Stepwise regression of	I	0.7017	0.4924	1086.396	0.000	In: PF	0.7017
General Health by	2	0.7616	0.5800	772.526	0.000	In: MH	0.3125
Physical Functioning,	3	0.7855	0.6171	600.551	0.000	In: LLI	− 0.2393
Mental Health, age,	4	0.7907	0.6252	465.754	0.000	In: SEX	− 0.0910
sex and LLI (final							
model)							

Multiple R	0.79068
R Square	0.62517
Adjusted R Square	0.62383
Standard Error	15.41411

Analysis of Variance

	DF	Sum of Squares	Mean Square
Regression	4	442642.74738	110660.68684
Residual	1117	265393.36993	237.59478
F = 465.75386		Signif F = 0.0000	

Variable	**B**	**SE B**	**95% Confdnce Intrvl B**		**Beta**
PF	0.378014	0.018702	0.341320	0.414709	0.472634
LLI	− 11.737170	1.145037	− 13.983835	− 9.490505	− 0.233598
SEX	− 4.585093	0.933705	− 6.417105	− 2.753080	− 0.090954
MH	0.411037	0.025953	0.360115	0.461958	0.308940
(Constant)	12.758811	2.350491	8.146936	17.370687	

There may be times when you require a variable to be in the model even though your friend the computer believes it is not adding anything to the model. You then have to decide whether to include this variable or not.

Another method of assessing the fit of a model is to examine the residuals. Are there many cases where the model appears to fit badly, and how many of these are there? In Table 10.12 we show an example of the some of the cases where the model does not seem to fit so well for the example in Table 10.10.

Table 10.12	**Code**	**Actual**	**Predicted**	**Residual**
Actual General Health	694	60.00	91.60	− 31.60
scores compared to	704	15.00	60.12	− 45.12
that predicted by	776	87.00	54.43	32.57
regression model in	820	45.00	77.60	− 32.60
Table 10.10 for some	935	90.00	50.53	39.47
of the outliers	946	15.00	62.37	− 47.37
	976	90.00	56.49	33.51
	1052	100.00	68.08	31.92
	1059	25.00	76.90	− 51.90
	1106	25.00	67.54	− 42.54
	1113	32.00	81.31	− 49.31
	1137	97.00	64.95	32.04
	1170	40.00	75.37	− 35.37
	1180	40.00	75.18	− 35.18

The predicted value from the equation is shown and the residual is calculated by subtracting the predicted from the actual score. There are more technical ways of analysing residuals, which we shall leave to more specialist textbooks, and also of deciding if a particular subject (respondent) has too great an influence on the final model. If one subject has too much influence, it is worth removing that subject from the analysis and re-running the regression to see how different the model would be without that subject.

10.4.4 Checking the validity of a model

You may have noticed that we have been a little lax so far in telling you the assumptions behind regression analysis. We will indicate briefly what this is all about, but this is where a trip to the statistician in your organization or the local university becomes necessary.

S/he will tell you that analysis of residuals tells us a lot about the validity of a model. For example, the residuals (observed minus expected – or predicted – values) should have an approximately normal distribution. Also, when plotted against the predicted values, there should be an even scattering, as in Figure 10.3(a), and not as in Figure 10.3(b), where the size of the residuals increases as the size of the predicted value increases.

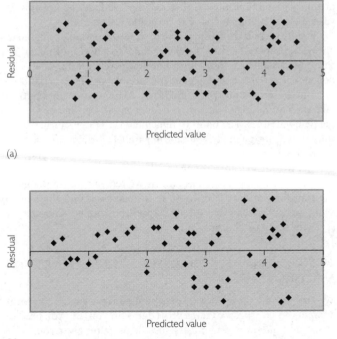

(a)

(b)

Predicted value

Predicted value

Figure 10.3

Scatterplots of predicted values against residuals. (a) Evenly scattered, no systematic deviation. (b) Increasing variability for higher values

A second issue is multicollinearity. This is where there is a high level of correlation between the independent variables. This is a problem we might have run into if we had used all the SF-36 scales as explanatory variables and it is a problem we have run into with age, since it is highly associated with LLI and PF. That is why age as an independent variable adds little to our model. Indeed, it is associated even with gender, since females tend to live longer. That is why it is recommended that you produce scatterplots of the independent variables against each other in order to see if any relationship reveals itself. If so, the best solution is probably careful selection of the variables, removing one of the correlated variables.

You may have noticed the 'Tolerance' and 'VIF' statistics in the SPSS output in Tables 10.9 and 10.10. The tolerance is used to determine the extent to which the independent variables are correlated to one another. If the tolerance is very low then problems arise in the calculation of the regression analysis and the results may be misleading. Related to this is the variance inflated factor (or VIF), which is the reciprocal of the tolerance (i.e. 1 divided by the tolerance). Some observers believe collinearity becomes a problem if the VIF statistic is 10 or above for any variable. Obviously, collinearity is not a problem for the simple linear regression case where there is only one independent variable.

A third problem is heteroscedascity. This occurs when the variance of the dependent variable is very different for different values of the independent variable. For example, older age groups might show much greater variability in their GH scores than younger age groups. If the variance is the same, it is said to be homoscedastic.

Finally there is the teasing issue of 'transformation', something that always appears rather like 'sleight of hand' to a non-statistician. Transforming variables can often turn non-linear relationships between the dependent variable and independent variable into linear relationships, or improve the validity of a model. A common transformation is to take the natural log of either the dependent and/or one or more independent variables. The point to remember is that the 'normal distribution' or 'regression models' are ideal 'parallel world' representations of the real world – necessary because mathematical laws function in this parallel world. So transforming real data so that it is in a form to which the maths can apply is fine, as long as we remember two things. First, the transformed data have to be re-formed back into the real world again. Second, whatever is done to the transformed data must make sense in 'real world' terms.

10.5 PROCEDURE FOR PERFORMING A LINEAR REGRESSION ANALYSIS

We will assume that you will use a computer package to perform the computational aspects of these procedures for you. But you need to ask it the right questions and understand the output it gives you.

(a) Decide whether linear regression analysis is the best method for meeting your objective. Remember, it assesses the linear relationship between variables and they may have a non-linear relationship.

(b) Produce scatterplots of the dependent variable against each of the independent variables and assess by eye the straight-line (linear) relationship between the variables.

(c) Assess the correlation between the independent variables by scatterplot and correlation coefficients; select the starting independent variables.

(d) Decide on method of entry into the model (if multiple regression); whether entering all the variables, selecting subsets of variables and comparing the models by the adjusted R^2 or using forward, backward or stepwise regression to select a subset of the variables.

(e) Assess the fit of the model by the value for R^2 (simple linear regression) or adjusted R^2 (multiple regression) and by assessing the residuals.

(f) Check for collinearity between the selected variables by looking at the tolerance and/or VIF and check the residuals for non-normality and plot them against the predicted values.

(g) Do not try to extrapolate beyond the range of your sample data. For example, if we used income as a variable and the highest income was £30 000 in our sample data, it would be unwise to try and predict for someone with an income of £60 000. We would then be assuming that our linear relationship holds outside the range of our data.

10.6 OTHER FORMS OF REGRESSION

There are many other forms of regression, which may be more appropriate but are outside the realms of this book. For example, in linear regression analysis we need the dependent variable to be of interval/ratio scale measurement. For a dichotomous (two category) dependent variable (such as having an LLI or not) we could use **logistic** regression. For occasions when we have categorical dependent and independent variables, such as from contingency tables, we would need to use **logit** modelling. For non-linear relationships we would need to use some other form of regression analysis depending on the type of relationship. One special case you may come across in the literature is based on a single independent variable but both the variable (X) and the square of the variable (X^2) are included in the model. This is a quadratic model and instead of a straight line (linear) relationship, the points when plotted should rise and then fall or fall and then rise.

10.7 A WORD ABOUT OUR CHOICE OF MODEL

The variables you select will have a major effect on your model. We have used in our example two of the scales on the SF-36, Physical Functioning and Mental Health, to help explain a third, General Health. These were chosen because they represent physical and mental health, respectively. However, we could have used other scales or all of them though this may lead to problems of multicollinearity. Using age, LLI and gender leads to age and LLI but not gender being selected by stepwise regression and 35% of the variance (based on the adjusted R^2) of GH being accounted for (compared to 62% in our model). Then adding MH to the model leads to all four variables being selected and 50% of the variance being accounted for. Removing MH and adding PF again leads to inclusion of all four variables and the adjusted R^2 jumping to 54%. As you can see, we cannot just leave the computer to decide but must firstly choose the variables we believe are practical, convenient and make common sense for inclusion into the model.

Regression analysis has been used in published studies of the SF-36 to remove the effects of factors like age and gender on the scale scores (Garratt, 1994; Lyons et al., 1994).

10.8 REGRESSION AND ANALYSIS OF VARIANCE

We mentioned at the end of the last chapter that regression analysis and analysis of variance were strongly related. The general factorial ANOVA command in SPSS for Windows even gives the regression coefficients and associated R^2 and adjusted R^2 values. Also, take a look at Table 10.13, produced within the simple factorial ANOVA command, performed only on the main effects and with age, Physical Functioning and Mental health as covariates (since they are interval/ratio scale data). Notice that we get the same p-value for age as in the regression analysis in Table 10.10, and its lack of significance is again highlighted.

Table 10.13	Source of Variation	Sum of Squares	DF	Mean Square	F	Sig of F
Analysis of variance of	Covariates					
General Health by	AGE	15.493	1	15.493	0.065	0.799
Physical Functioning,	PF	84758.400	1	84758.400	356.437	0.000
Mental Health, LLI,	MH	58250.420	1	58250.420	244.962	0.000
age and sex	Main Effects					
	LLI	24979.886	1	24979.886	105.049	0.000
	SEX	5716.505	1	5716.505	24.040	0.000
	Explained	442658.241	5	88531.648	372.304	0.000
	Residual	265377.877	1116	237.794		
	Total	708036.117	1121	631.611		

It is also possible in regression analysis to include the interaction terms we talked about when discussing ANOVAs in our model.

10.9 SUMMARY

In this chapter we have learnt about relationships between variables. Regression analysis is a complicated business and it is well worth seeking advice before and during attempting it. However, this chapter will hopefully have given you the ability to decide whether it is an appropriate technique for your data and how to interpret the output and start checking the validity of models created by your computer package. It will also help you read papers in journals that produce analysis by association and regression.

11 THE STATISTICS OF RANDOMIZED CONTROLLED TRIALS

11.1 THE CONTROLLED EXPERIMENT

A practice nurse runs an asthma clinic in a general practice. A new inhaler has been introduced and, with one of the practice doctors and one of the local chest physicians, she becomes involved in a study to evaluate how good the new inhaler might be. The next 10 patients to visit the asthma clinic are switched on to the new treatment. One month later seven of them say their breathing is better than before. 'Well, the new inhaler seems impressive' says the consultant at their next meeting.

Are you impressed? Or do you want to ask some questions? There are plenty to ask.

A first question might be: 'Would they have felt better anyway, despite the new inhaler?' Thinking of other things that might influence asthma symptoms, you might ask: Had they come to the clinic in the first place because colds or flu had made their asthma worse – when the infection got better, so did the asthma? Were they given other treatments, such as antibiotics or steroid tablets, which might have been the reason for their improvement? Did the weather change in the month on the new inhaler? Did the nurse, in taking time to explain the new inhaler, spend a lot more time than usual talking about other aspects of their asthma, which might have made this group of patients feel better? How did she talk about the new inhaler: e.g. did she say 'Here is something which might make you feel a lot better'? Suggestion is a very powerful treatment.

All these questions are directed at one issue. Were there other explanations for the improvements reported by the asthma patients than the idea that the new inhaler is an improvement on the old one? One way to answer this is to have a control group.

The study team realize this. They decide to expand their small pilot study and change another 20 patients on to the new inhaler. This time the nurse also picks 20 patients out who are not put on to the new inhaler but who are asked to come back in a month's time for assessment just like the group who get the new inhaler. At the end of this study, 17 patients on the new inhaler feel better, compared with 12 patients in the control group. 'Mmm. Even more impressive' says the enthusiastic consultant.

Are you impressed yet? More probably you are bursting with even more questions this time? How did the nurse pick the controls – were they the ones who were doing fine anyway and she did not wish to disturb their treatment? Were they older than the group who got the new inhaler? Were they the ones who did not really want to take part in the study once it was explained to them? Did the nurse still spend more time with the group who got the new treatment, and still give them the idea that it was going to be better than the old one?

In other words, you are concerned that there are other explanations for the different outcomes in the two groups than the fact that one group got the new inhaler and the other one did not.

The study team visits a statistician. The statistician breathes the magic words 'randomized controlled trial' and tells them to send her enough information so that she can calculate how big the study needs to be and to prepare a submission to the local ethics committee for approval. The team come up with a new idea.

Consecutive patients who come to the asthma clinic, and who are aged between 18 and 50 years, who are all on the same inhaler treatment and who have had no changes in the treatment for the past 3 months, will be told in detail about the study. Those who consent to be in the study will have a special assessment of their symptoms using a questionnaire and a meter that measures their breathing capacity. This will be administered by another practice nurse, specially trained for this task. The patients are then given a numbered envelope containing the inhaler that they will use for the next 4 weeks: the nurse records the number from the envelope on the patient's records. These envelopes contain one of two types of inhaler. These two inhalers look identical, but one type contains the new drug and one contains the old one. The numbers are the key to which patient has got which type of inhaler, and a master list to identify this is to be kept by the local pharmacist who made up the packages, as well as by the practice manager, for security. The envelopes have been prepared in a random order by the statistician, so the probability that any patient gets the new or the old treatment has been determined by the random number table and nothing else. One month later all the patients have a second assessment of their symptoms. The statistician compares the results between patients on the two treatments, using the patient's envelope number and the master list to allocate each patient to the appropriate group. The doctor, the asthma clinic nurse, the practice nurse brought in to do the assessments, and the patients themselves – none of them are aware of which treatment has been given to which patient.

You probably still have some questions to ask – you have got this far in the book after all, and your critical skills are red hot. But why do you feel more comfortable with this design? Mainly because strenuous attempts have been made to remove the effect of all other explanations for any differences that emerge between the two groups except for the one thing which you are interested in: namely that the two groups have received different treatments.

The controlled experiment lies at the heart of science. The simple argument is that if you can control everything in an environment to be the same and unchanging for the period of an experiment, and you then introduce one single factor for change, then any changes that subsequently occur can reasonably be attributed to that new factor. Since there was a stable situation beforehand, whatever you have introduced is assumed to be responsible for any subsequent differences.

11.2 THE RANDOMIZED CONTROLLED TRIAL

11.2.1 Features of the randomized controlled trial

In a world of real people and real illness, the 'scientific experiment' is difficult to achieve because people are living changing beings who cannot be 'controlled' in the same way that inanimate factors in a scientific experiment can be. In particular there are all sorts of unknown factors and influences on the physical and mental states of individuals that we cannot actually measure.

The answer to this problem has been the development of the randomized controlled trial. This form of experiment, which can be applied to people, to procedures or to institutions, is based on the following idea, illustrated by the example above.

(a) A group of patients is selected with a particular problem, the effect of a new treatment on which you wish to investigate.

(b) Each patient is allocated at random to one of two groups. The idea of allocating at random is based on the idea that you are giving each individual an equal chance of ending up in either of the two groups. At the end of the procedure, therefore, you hope that there will be equal numbers of older people, cigarette smokers, people who are anxious, people who are overweight, in each of the two groups. In other words in broad terms you have achieved a balance between the groups with respect to all sorts of characteristics which might also be linked to the condition that you are studying. In particular all those characteristics that you do not know about, but which are linked to the condition in question, or which you cannot measure but are linked to the condition in question, will also be balanced out.

(c) You give your intervention to one group but not to the other, and then you look at some measurable outcome 1 week or 1 month or 1 year later, and any difference in that outcome between the two groups you confidently attribute to your treatment. If there is no difference in the outcome you assume that your treatment has no effect on the condition.

11.2.2 Problems that might arise

The above all sounds very neat and tidy and scientific. There are two problems with it however.

- The first and most important is that there may be various ways in which bias can creep in, various ways in which the groups may surreptitiously become different, despite your careful planning. In the example above, suppose the new inhaler causes indigestion. The patients will soon latch on to this, and so will be aware that they are getting the new treatment; they may lower the dose because it is not so pleasant to use; and they may tell the assessing nurse about it so she will be aware that they have been on the new treatment and that anyone who comes in with indigestion is probably on the new treatment too. All of this may have an influence on the results.

We will consider some general points of possible bias in randomized controlled trials in the next section, not because they particularly involve statistical analysis but because we wish to emphasize that no statistical analysis in the world can cover up for an error in the study design that leads to bias, and because too often a statistical test is assumed to be the last word on whether a finding is true or not. The most important influence on truth, first and foremost, is to decide whether there was any bias in your study: are you comfortable that the only likely explanation for differences between the groups is that the intervention under investigation was different in the two groups?

- Assuming that you have managed to do the study without introducing too much in the way of bias, it remains possible that, despite your careful random allocation of individual patients to the two groups, by chance you have ended up with more smokers in one group than another, or more obese people in one group than another. The question then becomes: 'Might that difference be sufficient to have given you the results that you have got, quite separately to any effect of the treatment?' This would be bad news, because you would be attributing to the treatment a power and a potency that was in reality due to the groups in your experiment ending up by chance different in a certain crucial feature. Note how this is different from the bias that arises because of bad study design. Here you are actually attributing the difference to the ebb and flow of chance, the probability that in your experiment random allocation might end up with some differences existing between the groups.

It is in this context, and to address this particular problem, that statistics come into their own. Indeed it is one of the purest applications of probability statistics, to assess the role of chance in a randomized controlled trial, because you are saying 'given that I have used a random means to allocate patients to each of these two groups, what are the laws that govern this random allocation, which I can apply to assess how likely it is that chance alone has produced the observed result?'.

11.3 BRIEF OVERVIEW OF BIAS IN RANDOMIZED CONTROLLED TRIALS

There are a number of ways in which bias may arise. However it is important to be clear about the exact question that a randomized controlled trial wishes to ask before assuming that a particular procedure is biased or not. Let us take some variations on the asthma trial discussed earlier. For example, suppose the new inhaler is rather different to the old one in how it is used and patients will have to be taught how to use it. This rules out the idea that you can make the new treatment identical to the old one. The team leans towards a slightly different question and a different design: let us get a group of patients together whose control is less than ideal, and randomize them to receive the new inhaler or not to use it. One problem with this is that when the intervention group are called up to receive their inhaler, the 10 minutes that the nurse takes to explain how to use the new inhaler and its possible advantages and disadvantages would in itself be an extra intervention. On its own this might have an influence on how good asthma control becomes, since the other group are being deprived of this particular special consultation with the practice nurse.

The design team then goes back to the drawing board and say, OK, fine, what we will do is to send for all the patients with poor asthma control whom we might consider could benefit. We will explain to them all that there is a new treatment, but that we wish to do a study on it first, and for this trial we are asking people whether they would be willing to take a chance that they might be getting the active treatment (the real inhaler) or an inhaler that contains a harmless but inactive substance. Since you are going to ask all of the patients to continue to use whatever current treatment that they are on, in order to study whether there is added value from the new inhaler, you can reassure the patients that their usual treatment will be unaffected by being in the study. The practice nurse will carry out the same session for 10 minutes, explaining the new treatment and how it is used with both groups, regardless of whether the individuals are getting a real inhaler or the inactive inhaler. So in this trial design you are getting round the problem that the activities and intervention of the nurse might be as important as or more important than any effect of the new inhaler.

It is important to realize that both of these designs are valid but they depend on the question being asked. If you want to know whether the whole package (nurse, consultation plus inhaler) is effective in helping asthma the first design might be fine. If you feel the important question is to identify exactly whether the new inhaler had any additional effect because of the active drug it contains then the second design might be your choice. The first design is sometimes called a **pragmatic** trial, because it is taking into account how the whole package will be delivered in practice in primary care if it becomes the accepted treatment. The second type of design is sometimes called an **explanatory** trial, because it is looking at the narrower, but initially perhaps more important question of whether the new drug in the inhaler works better than current inhalers.

Imagine that you are the practice nurse in the explanatory trial described above, and you are aware which inhaler is the real one and which contains the inactive substance. Perhaps they look a little different for example. If you have read some literature about the new drug that has convinced you that this really will be of major benefit to your patients, there may be subtle influences on you when you are giving the advice to the patients. However much trialists believe that they can act in a completely independent fashion, many studies have shown that, if people are aware of the treatment that they are giving out, this awareness does influence the style and the way in which that treatment is delivered. This is a form of bias, because it may be that some of the advantages that you observe at the end of your study of the active inhaler are really attributable to the enthusiasm and the optimism which the practice nurse introduced at the start of the study because she was aware that she was prescribing the active inhaler to that group. This is sometimes called **investigator bias**.

Think now of the end of the study, and the questionnaire that perhaps will be used to judge the symptoms of the patients in the two groups 3 months after they were entered into the study. Thinking again of the explanatory trial, suppose it is the general practitioner who is asking the questions of the patients about their asthma control. Suppose once again that the doctor, like the nurse, knows which group the patient has been in and which treatment s/he has had. Once again bias may creep in because that knowledge may influence the way in which the questions are asked and the likelihood that positive or negative answers may be obtained. This is sometimes called **observer bias**.

The final possibility is that the patients themselves are aware of which treatment they have. As in our earlier version, suppose the inactive inhaler has a peculiar taste, which is exactly the same taste that the patients remember when they were being trained in the use of the inhaler when they first became asthmatic. This might lead the majority of them to guess that they were getting an inactive inhaler again. Once again, such awareness may influence the answers and the perceptions that they have about the control of their asthma symptoms. This is sometimes called **subject bias**.

In summary, we can see that there is a problem of awareness. One way in which trials get round this problem if they need to (because of the nature of the question being asked) is to ensure that the inactive treatment looks and tastes identical to the active treatment, and that both the nurse at the start and the doctor at the end are specifically excluded from knowledge of which is which. This is called **double blinding**, because both patient and the investigators have been kept unaware of which is which.

There is a second type of bias, which is rather different. In the course of the 3 months patients may get fed up with using the new inhaler (regardless of whether it is inactive or active) and stop using it. They may then subsequently not turn up to the follow-up appointment with the doctor where he is going to assess the control of the asthma. If there is a small dropout like this in both groups, and it has not been affected by whether they are getting active treatment or inactive treatment then this may not affect the final comparison. If, however, such drop out involves large numbers, and particularly if it is different in the two groups (e.g. perhaps there is a higher dropout in the group using the active inhaler because it has made them all sick) then there may well be a problem of **dropout bias**. If you only analyse the results of those who stay in the study and turn up for the follow-up, and if all those people who are being sick on the new inhaler choose not to turn up for that follow-up appointment because they feel rather angry and let down by the whole affair, then you may be presented with only half of your patients in the group on the active treatment. However it happens to be the half that were entirely happy with their treatment and indeed who did rather well on it who turn up. You may make the false deduction that it is a good treatment to use in primary care. It may be a good treatment for those people who do not react with the sickness, but overall it might be a rather ineffective treatment because half of the patients will develop the side effect.

This leads to an important principle in randomized controlled trials, that there are two types of analysis of the data that can be done. It is legitimate, particularly if your trial is very much concerned with trying to establish whether there is any effect of your new intervention or not (i.e. the explanatory trial), to analyse the results only of all those people who completed the treatments and presented back for the follow-up. However, presenting those results alone, as we have seen, may present a very biased picture of the truth, and so a second type of analysis (the 'intention to treat' type of analysis) is now accepted as being very important. This analysis includes everyone who was entered into the trial regardless of whether they stayed in until the end or not. There are of course problems with this in terms of getting adequate data on those who dropped out as to what their symptoms were like. However it emphasizes the need to get that sort of data even if people withdraw from the trial, and of considering what the possible effect may be if you assume that all the dropouts have not improved.

Table 11.1 illustrates an example of the two analyses in an example where weight reduction was being used in primary care as a treatment for hypertension in patients who were obese.

Table 11.1

Mean systolic blood pressure of all patients in hypertensive groups at entry, and at 6-month follow-up or point of dropout; and of those patients still attending after 6 months

	Mean systolic blood pressure (mmHg) (95% confidence interval)	
	Initial	Final
All initial attenders		
Hypertensive dieters ($n = 66$)	161 (157.5, 164.5)	150 (146.0, 154.0)
Hypertensive non-dieters ($n = 64$)	161 (157.5, 164.5)	157 (153.5, 160.5)
Patients attending after 6 months		
Hypertensive dieters ($n = 47$)	160 (156.1, 163.9)	147 (142.7, 151.3)
Hypertensive non-dieters ($n = 50$)	158 (155.4, 160.6)	155 (151.3, 158.7)

Some dropped out, but in those who persisted with the dieting the weight loss resulted in a fall in blood pressure. Overall weight reduction appeared to be effective, despite the dropout from the group during the 6 months follow-up. Both results are helpful, but they address different questions.

11.4 ANALYSIS OF RANDOMIZED CONTROLLED TRIALS

11.4.1 The null hypothesis

We considered the null hypothesis in Chapter 8 but revisit it here simply to point out its particular relevance to randomized controlled trials. One popular way to analyse trials from a statistical point of view is to present the actual difference between the two groups (e.g. the difference in severity of asthma scores between the two groups in our study described above), with a 95% confidence interval around that difference. For example 'the severity on the asthma scale was a mean of 2.0 higher in the inactive group compared with the group using the active inhaler, with a 95% confidence interval of 0.9–3.1 around that difference'. It is important to be clear whether that difference represents a clinically important difference (does a 2.0 difference in score mean easier breathing and a better life for the patient, for example?).

However there is another approach to analysis that is particularly suitable to the whole issue of randomized controlled trials. The approach is to say that one is looking for the probability that the difference that you observe in any randomized controlled trial has arisen by chance, i.e. it has arisen as a result of the randomization. The starting point for this calculation is to make the assumption that there is no difference between the groups in truth, in other words that the difference between any mean scores or median ratings and so on is zero. This is the null hypothesis.

Any particular trial that is comparing two groups between which the true difference is zero will be more or less close to that zero, depending on the extent of random error in that particular trial. So the smaller the trial, for example, the higher the probability that a result that is different from zero may have arisen by chance, when the truth is that the difference is truly zero. If the next sample examining the same question is much larger, then the probability this time that a result has arisen by chance will be rather lower. The tests of statistical significance described in earlier chapters, which are based on t-tests for mean scores or the chi-square for frequencies, can be applied in this situation to the observed difference between groups in a randomized controlled trial. The probability that is calculated, on the usual basis of the size of the observed difference, the size of the sample and the standard deviation or variance of the difference between the groups, represents in the randomized controlled trial the exact probability that the result that you have observed might have arisen by chance. As in earlier examples the conventional cut off for considering that a difference is 'statistically significantly different from zero' is a probability value less than 0.05.

The main drawback of the null hypothesis approach in trials is that it focuses on the black-and-white issues: has the intervention had an effect or not? 'The new inhaler resulted in an improvement in asthma severity score statistically significantly different to placebo, $p < 0.05$.' This is clear and, if the trial was free of bias, convincing. But it does not tell us how big the improvement was, and how important that improvement might be for asthmatics to have. Such questions cannot be answered by the p-value alone.

11.4.2 Relative measures of effect

Important as the null hypothesis and the p-value are to the analysis of the randomized controlled trial, health services research has shifted its focus to other estimates of effect.

Let us take an example from the meta-analysis literature. We briefly described the meta-analysis in Chapter 3. It involves a systematic selection from all studies on a particular topic, based on their quality, and an attempt to statistically pool the results of all those that reach certain minimum criteria of freedom from bias. An article from the *British Journal of General Practice* (Williamson and Whelan, 1996) reviewed results from trials of steroid therapy in the treatment of facial palsy, an acute paralysis that can be slow to recover completely. This overview concluded that the complete recovery rate in patients who received steroid treatment was 77% after 1 year compared to 68% in those who had received control treatments. This pooled result was statistically significantly different from the null hypothesis of no difference between the treatment groups ($p = 0.03$).

The two figures in the last paragraph can be compared in other ways.

First a ratio can be calculated. The steroid groups were overall 77 / 68 times more likely to improve compared with the controls, i.e. there was a **relative benefit** of 1.13 or 13%. (If we were dealing with an adverse outcome such as death, then the term used would be the more familiar **relative risk** or **risk ratio**.) This benefit ratio or relative benefit can be presented with a 95% confidence interval: in the published pooled data, this was 1–27%.

An alternative to the relative benefit or risk is the **odds ratio**. This is popular because of its ease of analysis in a type of regression called logistic regression, based on a dichotomous outcome (full recovery versus partial or no recovery in this instance). 'Odds' are intuitively more difficult to grasp than the proportions indicated by risk or benefit, but the interpretation is similar.

Odds of full recovery on steroids = 77:23 = 3.4:1.

In other words, the two sides of odds do not contain each other. Out of every 100 patients on steroids, 77 recover fully and 23 do not, i.e. for every 1 person who does not recover on steroids, 3.4 do recover. Compare this to the proportional benefit (or risk)

Likelihood of full recovery on steroids = 77 / 100 = 77%.

The denominator (all 100 patients given steroids) includes the numerator (the 77 who recover) this time; in other words, out of 100 people who receive steroids, 77 recover.

The odds ratio compares the odds of full recovery on steroids with the odds of full recovery on control therapies. It represents the association of steroid therapy with full recovery

Odds of full recovery on control therapies = 68:32 = 2.1:1
Odds ratio = 3.4 / 2.1 = 1.6.

So the odds that people on steroids will recover fully is 1.6 higher than the odds that people on control therapy will recover fully. Note that odds ratios tend to be higher than relative benefit or relative risks.

11.4.3 Absolute measures of effect

The odds ratio is calculated for statistical convenience. More important than the odds ratio and the relative benefit or risk is the absolute benefit. This is the actual proportion of patients who recover on steroids, over and above the proportion who would recover on control therapy.

Absolute benefit = 77% – 68% = 9%

The interpretation is that, out of 100 people on steroid treatment, nine more have recovered than would have done if they had been on control treatment. It is a measure of the actual benefit that might be expected from switching everyone on to steroids rather than using the control treatment. Again, confidence intervals can be placed around this figure. The importance of this measure is that you can relate it to how common the problem is. If, for example, 1000 patients are going to be seen in primary care with facial palsy, 680 patients will recover whatever treatment you choose. But if all 1000 go on to steroid therapy, an extra 90 will recover as well. The relative benefit (770 / 680 = 1.13 = 13%) is still the same whether we were considering 100 or 1000 patients, i.e. whatever the total number treated. Absolute figures can be used to help in judging the overall benefits and costs of treatment strategies.

A final way to get insight into the implications of randomized controlled trials is 'the number needed to treat'. Among 100 patients treated with steroids, it is estimated that there are nine whose recovery has been hastened because they were on steroids rather than control treatment. This reduces down to the statement that there is one extra recovery for every 11 patients on steroids. This is then put as '11 patients must be treated with steroids for one additional patient to recover completely'. This number needed to treat provides another perspective to help actual decision making, and once again confidence intervals can be calculated for this figure: in the article the pooled interval was 6–117.

11.5 Summary

In summary, randomized controlled trials are powerful means to investigate the effect of interventions by ensuring that the effects of other factors will only arise by chance. The likelihood that any differences have arisen by chance is expressed by the p-value. The size of the benefit or risk of an intervention can be summarized by relative measures such as benefit or risk ratios or by odds ratios. The actual size of any benefit is best expressed by absolute or interval differences, and by 'number needed to treat'. The influence of chance on these summaries can all be indicated by 95% confidence intervals.

And finally, remember that statistics are not a judge of truth. Bias in a randomized trial will be removed not by statistics but by good design.

12 WRITING UP AND DISSEMINATION

12.1 INTRODUCTION

Writing up your research tends to be seen as the last big job to be done on a project. Yet it should be thought about right from the start because the way in which you report relates directly to the audience and users of your findings. Increasingly, research funders will stipulate at the outset what they expect in terms of output and lay that down within written agreements or formal contracts. This means that you are immediately focused on the product you have to deliver at the end of your research and this influences how you analyse the data – or at least how you think about alternative approaches.

In this chapter we discuss the most common forms of presenting your findings: the written research report for funders can take many guises ranging from a detailed scientific report to a set of recommendations; feedback to participants in the study, often lay people who would like to know the broad findings; articles for academic journals or professional publications; oral presentations. The question of dissemination of findings is becoming more important because research has demonstrated that just publicizing findings through the traditional sources does not necessarily mean that they are taken up and implemented in practice (Lomas and Haynes, 1988). We will therefore also touch upon this issue and offer some suggestions.

12.2 WHAT TO WRITE FOR WHICH TARGET AUDIENCE?

12.2.1 The research report

A written report is almost always required at the end of a research project, but the form this takes varies depending on the target audience. We outline the main principles of good report writing and indicate where there are differences depending on who the report goes to and what it will be used for.

In general a report begins with an executive summary setting out the purpose of the study, how the research was designed and carried out, highlighting the key findings and presenting the conclusion. This summary should indeed be a summary, i.e. concise and limited in length (two to three A4 pages).

The main body of the report should start with an introduction that clearly states the research question or hypothesis, the background to the research and the structure of the report.

The next section focuses on the methodology adopted and this can vary in detail, but should at the minimum describe the research design, the population studied, the main measurement tools adopted and the analytical methods, and why they were selected. The informed lay audience, e.g. Health Authority managers who have asked you to carry out a health needs assessment, will find this level of reporting adequate because it provides them with a clear impression of the robustness of the approach without going into the intricacies of design and analysis. They are primarily interested in the outcomes and recommendations but want to be assured that the research underpinning those is of an acceptable quality.

An academic audience will want a scientific report where considerable detail is required. This pertains to the following areas in particular: the justification for the study population; the criteria for inclusion or exclusion from the study population, which should be spelled out; and the way in which the sample was selected and assigned to groups (if appropriate).

If established measurement tools are adopted, like the SF-36 in our example, then it is important to explain why you chose this measure and to provide a critical review of the literature. This will help to assess the robustness of the tool because other studies can demonstrate the reliability and validity of the particular measure, or highlight any weaknesses that should be taken into account. Furthermore, through a comparative analysis of tools you are able to develop your argument as to why your choice of particular tools is appropriate to the purpose of the research. You also need to discuss the data collection strategy and how this is consistent with the methods adopted in the literature; or, where it is different, give the reasons for any diversion.

Should you decide to develop your own measurement tool for your research project you have a more difficult reporting task on your hands (apart from the considerable effort in actually undertaking the research). You need to justify the choice of developing your own tool by reviewing available alternatives, clearly illustrating their strengths and weaknesses. You then have to report on the various developmental stages of piloting, testing, re-testing and arriving at a reliable, validated tool. This is, of course, a less common approach and we will focus on the use of accepted tools.

The final part of the methodology section in a scientific report concerns the analysis. It is necessary to clearly explain the various methods used to test hypotheses or answer each research question, also justifying the choices you have made. For example, you need to state that in order to compare men and women on the different dimensions of the SF-36 you used the two-sample t-test. You can also mention here the levels of significance adopted or any other conventions that are relevant to your analysis.

Most readers will find the results section the most important part and it is important to make this easily readable and digestible. You will, of course, have more material than you can report and it is vital that you select judiciously with the target audience in mind. This generally means going back to the main hypotheses or questions and decide which ones your audience will require. In order to judge the results properly some basic information has first to be provided in terms of response rates, descriptive characteristics of the sample (e.g. sex, age, electoral ward, marital status, etc.) and any reservations about the accuracy of the data. You can then present your data with the reader in mind. Take your Health Authority manager, again, who is interested in the allocation of resources according to localities. For this person the results of the SF-36 scores broken down by locality will be most interesting. You can do this in tabular form using, for example, mean scale scores by ward for the people in the LLI group, including the *p*-values. However, a more user-friendly way could be to provide a graph that provides a quick visual overview of the differences (Figure 12.1).

Figure 12.1

Mean Short Form-36 scale scores by electoral ward for the LLI group.

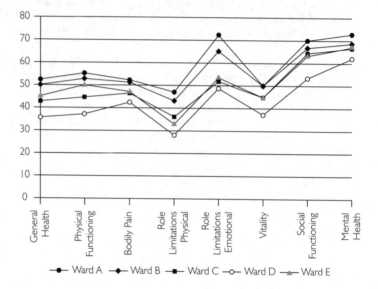

This type of information is easier to interpret for the person who wants to know whether there are differences in health status between localities, and in what areas as measured by the SF-36 in particular. Often you will be asked to provide tables as well because they are considered to provide more information and to be less easy to 'manipulate'.

Looking towards your academic audience, they will want more sophisticated analyses, such as comparing component scores across the wards. The SF-36 allows for a physical component summary score (PCS) to be calculated and a mental summary score (MCS). These component scores include all SF-36 scales, but they are 'weighted' more towards the physical and mental dimensions respectively. You can then present a table such as Table 12.1.

In most quantitative studies the presentation of the analysis is separate from the discussion, which offers an interpretation of the findings and commonly makes comparisons with other reported studies in the same field. The emphasis is on the critical assessment of your own findings and how they stand up against the available literature. It is also important to discuss any possible reservations you have about your own findings, e.g. because of low response rates or a high number of invalid responses.

			PCS		MCS	
		n	Mean (SD)	Median	Mean (SD)	Median
Total	LLI	501	43.4 (9.5)	42.4	48.2 (10.8)	49.9
	Non-LLI	553	56.0 (5.8)	57.1	51.7 (8.9)	54.3
Female 18–64	LLI	149	44.4 (9.8)	43.9	46.8 (12.1)	48.8
	Non-LLI	219	56.8 (5.6)	57.7	50.0 (10.0)	53.2
Female 65+	LLI	129	41.2 (8.1)	40.1	47.6 (9.7)	48.1
	Non-LLI	72	53.0 (7.1)	54.4	52.9 (7.0)	54.3
Male 18–64	LLI	137	45.0 (10.2)	43.3	49.0 (11.0)	52.5
	Non-LLI	195	56.7 (5.2)	57.3	52.4 (8.6)	55.2
Male 65+	LLI	86	42.5 (9.1)	41.6	50.0 (9.4)	50.8
	Non-LLI	67	54.5 (5.6)	56.2	53.6 (6.7)	55.3

Table 12.1

Component summary scores of the Short Form-36 by age and sex

PCS = physical component summary score; MCS = mental component summary score

It seems obvious, but you must continually ask yourself the question of why you want to present a particular part of your analysis and how it contributes to the overall picture you are trying to paint. It is no use swamping the audience with masses of data because they will lose sight of the key argument you are constructing. Thus, the presentation of your analysis has to relate directly to the discussion of the findings and the purpose of the research. Coming back to our example, the Health Authority manager wants to have evidence of whether there are differences between localities and the nature of those differences to help in making decisions about possible differential allocation of resources. The academic researcher is interested in issues such as the originality of your research, whether and how it contributes to existing knowledge, what can be learned from your design and methodology or the extent to which your study can be replicated. Therefore, the differences lie not only in the detail but also in the conceptual depth of the discussion. It is difficult to provide hard and fast rules as it is a question of 'being in touch' with your target audience. In the case of commissioned work, checking against the agreed contract is the best guideline to follow (and hopefully it is explicit about the end product!).

Every good report ends with a conclusion drawing together the main points of the report and outlining whether and how the key research questions were answered, or whether the main hypotheses were accepted or rejected. It is useful to briefly comment on how this study compares with other similar ones and whether new insights have been gained. The limitations of your study have to be touched upon, which often leads to the final conclusion that more research needs to be done (this is the conclusion in 90% of research reports!).

When you do research for funders who want to use your findings to influence policy and practice you tend to be asked to make recommendations. Your Health Authority manager falls into this category of users. So you have to answer questions such as: What do the differences in health status as measured by the SF-36 mean? What implications do these differences have for the allocation of resources to different localities? In order to make recommendations you probably have to refer to policy papers such as the organization's strategy. Should this explicitly state that the Health Authority wants to tackle inequalities in health you can recommend that, if the differences between localities are due to unequal access to health care, resources should be diverted to the most needy localities.

You must pay sufficient attention to the use of appendices. They should not be enormous, but provide essential information about the tools used (e.g. provide a full copy of the SF-36 questionnaire), the letters sent to respondents, informed consent forms used and any complicated calculations that would have made the main body of the report difficult to read, but which are essential to the analysis. For an academic report a full reference list has to be appended using one of the two main reference systems, Harvard or Vancouver.

Fink (1993) offers a very useful checklist against which a research report can be judged (her list is most appropriate for evaluation research, but it contains sufficient general principles to be relevant for the type of studies discussed in this book).

12.2.2 The academic paper

There are a various types of academic paper, including the conference paper, book chapter, occasional paper (produced by university departments), article for an academic journal using a refereeing system. We focus on the last as the standards are most rigorous for this type of paper. At the same time it is important to balance scientific credibility against coverage and we will deal with this question later on in this chapter.

Most of what we said about the academic report pertains to the academic paper, but the main difference is that you have less space in which to do the same job. The main decision you have to make is one of focus and that means segmenting your material. In the case of our LLI study we were able to divide it up into at least four papers: one reporting on the Census material and the LLI question, one on the SF-36 study, one on the comparison of the LLI and SF-36 results and general practice (GP) consultation, one on the total study, including the qualitative interviews. In order to be able to segment you need to choose the right journal for submission.

Almost every academic journal offers a statement of its aims and scope: there are journals that define their remit widely by accepting multidisciplinary research in the area of health policy and health services research; others focus in a narrower range and state, for example, that they are interested in statistical studies in the health care field only. Whatever the aims are it is vitally important that you assess whether your planned paper falls within the framework of a particular journal. Papers will be rejected if they fall outside the scope of the journal. Taking our LLI study, the paper on GP consultation was submitted to a medical journal while the one reporting the whole study went to a social science journal.

The second step is to study the guidelines for authors, which tend to explain how manuscripts have to be presented. It helps if you follow those guidelines to the letter because it makes a good impression and saves a lot of time later on when your paper is (hopefully) accepted. The main conventions are similar to the ones discussed above in relation to report writing, i.e. providing an abstract (generally only 200–300 words), key words (this is becoming increasingly important with the growth of computerized databases), statement of the objectives of your research, design and methods adopted, results, discussion, conclusion, references and any essential tables or figures. Copyright and conflict of interest statements are commonly requested.

Because the academic paper is much shorter in length (generally between 2000 and 8000 words in length) it is important to decide on a clear focus for your paper and as a result to be selective about the data you are going to use. Many journals stipulate a maximum number of tables and figures, forcing the writer to distinguish between the essential and the peripheral. Again, you must think about the user-friendliness of your presentation, in terms of both the clarity of your writing and the way in which you display your data.

Thinking about how the quality of papers is now being assessed through the mechanism of systematic reviews, it is useful to keep a number of questions in mind that help you to judge how your own product stands up. Greenhalgh (1997a) offers the following questions:

- Was the study original? Does this study add to the literature in any way, and how?
- Whom is the study about? How were subjects recruited, who was included/excluded, were subjects studied in real-life situations or not?
- Was the design of the study sensible? Did it fit with the stated objective? In the case of research trials questions need to be asked such as: What specific intervention was studied and what was it compared with? What outcome as measured, and how?
- Was systematic bias avoided or minimized, and how?
- Was the study large enough, or continued long enough, to make the results credible?

Answering these questions convincingly will go a long way in determining whether your paper is worth submitting to a journal.

12.2.3 The professional journal

The status of academic papers tends to be high within the scientific community because they are subjected to peer review. However, the coverage of these journals is variable, with the international journals enjoying the widest readership but some of the more specialist journals being read by a small group. The reporting of applied research often calls for several audiences, particularly including policy-makers and practitioners. The main consideration is that these are the people who can influence the dissemination of new ideas and the uptake of specific recommendations. Professional journals, or even mass media, could prove to be better vehicles than academic journals.

As with academic journals you need to investigate the aims and scope of the professional journals: some are unidisciplinary, e.g. nursing journals; others are focused on health policy and current debates. The style of the journals is another important factor to take into account as they can range from semiacademic to 'popular', determining what you put into an article and which tone you adopt. For academic researchers it is often very difficult to adjust to a more journalistic style of writing, but many journals edit articles to conform to their house style. You need to provide copy that falls squarely within their area of interest, written in an accessible (jargon-free) style and with user-friendly supporting evidence. Fink (1993) provides good examples of this approach: instead of using the phrase 'We established concurrent validity by correlating scores on Measure A with those on Measure B' she suggests 'We examined the relationship between the scores on Measures A and B' (p. 169).

12.2.4 Writing for the lay person

It is considered good practice to provide feedback to subjects of research, particularly if people have actively participated through answering questionnaires or being interviewed. While they generally do not want lengthy reports, they do like to know what the key results of the research projects are. The art of written feedback is to find a balance between reporting scientifically underpinned results and accessibility to an audience that varies in both degree of interest and education.

The solution we adopted in our LLI study was to write a one-page letter to respondents, highlighted the main findings and offering them the opportunity to request the main report. In our experience (in this study and previous ones) approximately 10% of subjects ask for a full report, with the remainder appearing to be happy with a letter. Other methods could include a short newspaper article or radio item, feedback via patient organizations (in the UK the Community Health Council is an appropriate vehicle) or other specific interest groups. If the study was carried out for a health organization their own communication channels, such as regular newsletters, could be used.

12.3 OTHER FEEDBACK METHODS

An oral presentation for the research funders is commonly part of the feedback process. Generally, the oral presentation is for key people within the organization and is used to support the written report. It is rare that it is the only way in which the research findings are made public.

Because the oral presentation is linked to a written report it is important to think carefully about its purpose. Is it solely to highlight key findings that people then look up in the report? Does it intend to change people's thinking about an issue and implement any recommendations? The purpose determines the emphasis within the presentation, e.g. a detailed account of the research design and analysis for an in-depth discussion of the findings, or a brief report on the research process with a more lengthy treatment of its implications.

The normal conventions of a good talk apply: the use of visual aids, which are clearly laid out and attractively produced; supporting handouts; a well-paced presentation discussing the objectives of the research, main methods, results, conclusions and recommendations (taking into account the question of balance discussed above); space for questions and comments; and some humour to keep people's attention.

12.4 THE QUESTION OF DISSEMINATION

In the health care field in many developed countries increasing attention has been directed towards effectiveness and cost-effectiveness. As part of this policy thrust the development of evidence-based care has been widely promoted, and the use of knowledge to improve the quality of health care –including health outcomes– forms an integral element of this 'movement'. Dissemination is a key concept, which can be defined in a number of ways: 'The spread of knowledge from its source to health care practitioners. It includes any special efforts to ensure that practitioners acquire a working acquaintance with that knowledge. Successful dissemination requires both accurate communication from the source and accurate understanding by the recipients ('competence')' (Lomas and Haynes, 1988, p. 77). The definition used by Kanouse *et al.* (1995) specifies the above in more detail: 'Dissemination ...is a process of communicating information that originates from one or more sources (biomedical research teams, NIH panels, professionals associations), is transmitted through various media (journals, conferences, word of mouth, popular press) and reaches various audiences (policy-makers, health care providers, payers, consumers)' (p. 168).

While you will be unlikely to be directly involved in all the processes, and in particular the social and educational processes, the task for the researcher reporting on the statistically based findings is important. If you are going to succeed in influencing the use of knowledge your reporting has to be relevant, transparent, succinct and integrated within a practice-oriented framework. Thus, when writing up the results of, for example, RCTs, the statistical side needs to clearly underpin the overall argument weighing up the strengths and weaknesses of the interventions that are compared, and be focused rather than offering a panoply of complicated calculations. Similarly, in health services research, policy-makers and planners want to know that the findings are robust, but can make do with a few – often simplified– tables and graphs illustrating whether, for example, there are significant differences in health status between localities. For you, the question of dissemination poses the challenge of presenting your statistical evidence in a manner that illuminates rather than confuses the reader and that is explicitly presented to underpin the broader clinical or policy argument. The same goes for when you have to present your findings verbally. Your words and supporting visual aids need to be geared towards the issue of whether the audience can grasp the importance of the statistical evidence and how it will help them to be convinced of the overall arguments or recommendations.

12.5 CONCLUSION

We have given you some straightforward ideas about the presentation of your material and the way in which it needs to be 'fit for purpose'. It is important to have a clear perspective on the purpose of your presentation and the target audience. Once those are defined you can tailor the way in which you will report on your findings. We hope that you yourself are less frightened about statistics, having read this book, so do not make others frightened in turn by obtuse reporting!

Appendix A
USEFUL WORLD WIDE WEB ADDRESSES

A.1 STATISTICAL COMPUTER SOFTWARE

Arcus Quickstat
http://www.camcode.com/

Epi Info
http://www.cdc.gov/epo/epi/epiinfo.htm

Microsoft Corporation (producers of the Excel spreadsheet within Microsoft Office)
http://www.microsoft.com/

MINITAB
http://www.minitab.com/

NCSS (Number Cruncher Statistical Software)
http://www.ncss.com/

SPSS (Statistical Package for the Social Sciences)
http://www.spss.com/

A.2 MISCELLANEOUS

Centre for Applied Social Surveys at the University of Surrey
http://www.soc.surrey.ac.uk/socresonline/2/2/cass.html

Centre for Applied Social Surveys Question Bank
http://kennedy.soc.surrey.ac.uk/qb/

Centre for Health Planning and Management, Keele University
http://www.keele.ac.uk/depts/hm/chpmhmpg.htm

Community Health Research Centre, Keele University
http://www.keele.ac.uk/depts/pm/chrc.htm

Short Form-36 (SF-36) home page
http://www.sf-36.com/

Stanley Thornes Publishing
http://www.thornes.co.uk/

UK Census details from Manchester Information Datasets and Associated Services (MIDAS) based at the University of Manchester
http://midas.ac.uk/census/census.html

Appendix B

STATISTICAL TABLES

Standard score	Percentile	Standard score	Percentile
– 2.3	1.1	0.1	54.0
– 2.0	2.3	0.2	57.9
– 1.9	2.9	0.3	61.8
– 1.8	3.6	0.4	65.5
– 1.7	4.5	0.5	69.2
– 1.6	5.5	0.6	72.6
– 1.5	6.7	0.7	75.8
– 1.4	8.1	0.8	78.8
– 1.3	9.7	0.9	81.6
– 1.2	11.5	1.0	84.1
– 1.1	13.6	1.1	86.4
– 1.0	15.9	1.2	88.5
– 0.9	18.4	1.3	90.3
– 0.8	21.2	1.4	91.9
– 0.7	24.2	1.5	93.3
– 0.6	27.4	1.6	94.5
– 0.5	30.9	1.7	95.5
– 0.4	34.5	1.8	96.4
– 0.3	38.2	1.9	97.1
– 0.2	42.1	2.0	97.7
– 0.1	46.0	2.3	98.9
0.0	50.0	3.0	99.9

For example, a standard score of – 1.4 equates to approximately the eighth percentile. A standard score of 1.4 equates to approximately the 92nd percentile.

z	α	z	α
0.000	1.00	1.282	0.20
0.126	0.90	1.645	0.10
0.253	0.80	1.960	0.05
0.385	0.70	2.326	0.02
0.524	0.60	2.576	0.01
0.674	0.50	2.807	0.005
0.842	0.40	3.291	0.001
1.036	0.30	3.891	0.0001

For example, a value for the Z statistic (z) of 1.96 equates to a significance level (α) of 0.05 or 5%. A value for the Z statistic (z) of 2.45 equates to a significance level (α) of between 0.02 and 0.01 (between 2% and 1%).

Degrees of freedom	$\alpha = 0.1$	$\alpha = 0.05$	$\alpha = 0.02$	$\alpha = 0.01$	$\alpha = 0.001$
1	6.314	12.706	31.821	63.657	636.619
2	2.920	4.303	6.965	9.925	31.599
3	2.353	3.182	4.541	5.841	12.924
4	2.132	2.776	3.747	4.604	8.610
5	2.015	2.571	3.365	4.032	6.869
6	1.943	2.447	3.143	3.707	5.959
7	1.895	2.365	2.998	3.499	5.408
8	1.860	2.306	2.896	3.355	5.041
9	1.833	2.262	2.821	3.250	4.781
10	1.812	2.228	2.764	3.169	4.587
11	1.796	2.201	2.718	3.106	4.437
12	1.782	2.179	2.681	3.055	4.318
13	1.771	2.160	2.650	3.012	4.221
14	1.761	2.145	2.624	2.977	4.140
15	1.753	2.131	2.602	2.947	4.073
16	1.746	2.120	2.583	2.921	4.015
17	1.740	2.110	2.567	2.898	3.965
18	1.734	2.101	2.552	2.878	3.922
19	1.729	2.093	2.539	2.861	3.883
20	1.725	2.086	2.528	2.845	3.850
21	1.721	2.080	2.518	2.831	3.819
22	1.717	2.074	2.508	2.819	3.792
23	1.714	2.069	2.500	2.807	3.768
24	1.711	2.064	2.492	2.797	3.745
25	1.708	2.060	2.485	2.787	3.725
30	1.697	2.042	2.457	2.750	3.646
40	1.684	2.021	2.423	2.704	3.551
50	1.676	2.009	2.403	2.678	3.496
60	1.671	2.000	2.390	2.660	3.460
70	1.667	1.994	2.381	2.648	3.435
80	1.664	1.990	2.374	2.639	3.416
90	1.662	1.987	2.368	2.632	3.402
100	1.660	1.984	2.364	2.626	3.390
∞	1.645	1.960	2.326	2.576	3.291

Table B3

Values of the t-distribution – two-tailed

For example, a value for the t-statistic of 2.447 on 6 degrees of freedom equates to a significance level (α) of 0.05 or 5%. A value for the t-statistic of 2.45 on 11 degrees of freedom equates to a significance level (α) of between 0.05 and 0.02 (between 5% and 2%).

Appendix B

Table B4

Values of the chi-squared (χ^2) distribution – two-tailed

Degrees of freedom	$\alpha = 0.1$	$\alpha = 0.05$	$\alpha = 0.02$	$\alpha = 0.01$	$\alpha = 0.001$
1	2.706	3.841	5.412	6.635	10.827
2	4.605	5.991	7.824	9.210	13.815
3	6.251	7.815	9.837	11.345	16.268
4	7.779	9.488	11.668	13.277	18.465
5	9.236	11.070	13.388	15.086	20.517
6	10.645	12.592	15.033	16.812	22.457
7	12.017	14.067	16.622	18.475	24.322
8	13.362	15.507	18.168	20.090	26.125
9	14.684	16.919	19.679	21.666	27.877
10	15.987	18.307	21.161	23.209	29.588
11	17.275	19.675	22.618	24.725	31.264
12	18.549	21.026	24.054	26.217	32.909
13	19.812	22.362	25.472	27.688	34.528
14	21.064	23.685	26.873	29.141	36.123
15	22.307	24.996	28.259	30.578	37.697
16	23.542	26.296	29.633	32.000	39.252
17	24.769	27.587	30.995	33.409	40.790
18	25.989	28.869	32.346	34.805	42.312
19	27.204	30.144	33.687	36.191	43.820
20	28.412	31.410	35.020	37.566	45.315
21	29.615	32.671	36.343	38.932	46.797
22	30.813	33.924	37.659	40.289	48.268
23	32.007	35.172	38.968	41.638	49.728
24	33.196	36.415	40.270	42.980	51.179
25	34.382	37.652	41.566	44.314	52.620

For example, a value for the χ^2 statistic of 12.592 on 6 degrees of freedom equates to a significance level (α) of 0.05 or 5%. A value for the χ^2-statistic of 21.03 on 11 degrees of freedom equates to a significance level (α) of between 0.05 and 0.02 (between 5% and 2%).

Appendix C
THE SHORT FORM-36 (SF–36)

The SF-36 (Ware *et al.*, 1993) is a health profile tool consisting of 36 questions. The questions can be grouped into scales relating to eight different dimensions of health – General Health (5 questions), Physical Functioning (10), Bodily Pain (2), Role Limitations due to Physical Problems (4), Role Limitations due to Emotional Problems (3), Vitality/Energy (4), Social Functioning (2) and Mental Health (5).

There is one question, which is unscaled, relating to change in health over the previous year.

Each of the answers for each question on a health scale are given scores. For each respondent, the scores for the answers for that scale are summed and then transformed to give a score on each health scale ranging from 0 (worst health) up to 100 (best health).

The SF-36 has an anglicized version to make some of the wording more familiar for a British setting. This is commonly known as the UK SF-36 and more details are given in Jenkinson *et al.*, 1996.

'SF-36' is a trademark of the Medical Outcomes Trust and anyone wishing to use the SF-36 should contact:

The Medical Outcomes Trust
20 Park Plaza
Suite 1014
Boston, MA 02116
USA.

The most common SF-36 asks respondents to recall their health over the previous 4 weeks, although there is also an acute, 1-week recall version. There are also shorter versions of the SF-36: the SF-6 and the SF-12. Details can be obtained either by writing to the Medical Outcomes Trust or via the home page for the SF-36 on the World Wide Web (see Appendix A).

REFERENCES

Allen, I. (ed.) (1993) *Rationing of health and social care*, Policy Studies Institute, London.

Altman, D. (1991) *Practical Statistics for Medical Research*, Chapman & Hall, London.

Altman, D. (1996) Use of confidence intervals to indicate uncertainty in research findings. *Evidence-Based Medicine*, **May/June**, 102–104.

Altman, D., Gore, S., Gardner, M. and Pocock, S. (1983) Statistical guidelines for contributors to medical journals. *British Medical Journal*, **286**, 1489–1493.

Baker, M. (1991) *Research for Marketing*, Macmillan, London.

Banta, H. D. and Vondeling, H. (1994) Strategies for successful evaluation and policy-making toward health care technology on the move: the case of medical lasers. *Social Science and Medicine*, **38**(12), 1663–1674.

Barnett, V. (1991) *Sample Survey Principles and Methods*, Edward Arnold, Sevenoaks.

Barriball, K., Christian, S., While, A. and Bergen, A. (1996) The telephone survey method – a discussion paper. *Journal of Advanced Nursing*, **24**, 115–121.

Bebbington, A. C. (1988) The expectation of life without disability in England and Wales. *Social Science and Medicine*, **27**, 321–326.

Begg, C. and Berlin, J. (1988) Publishing bias: a problem in interpreting medical data. *Journal of the RSS, Series A*, **151**, 419–463.

Benzeval, M. and Judge, K. (1993) *The 1991 Census Health Question*. Discussion Paper, King's Fund Institute, London.

Benzeval, M., Judge, K. and Whitehead, M. (eds) (1995) *Tackling Inequalities in Health: An Agenda for Action*, King's Fund, London.

Biles, C. (1995) *Statistics: A Health Sciences Orientation*, Wm. C. Brown, Dubuque, IO.

Bland, M. (1995) *An Introduction to Medical Statistics*, Oxford University Press, Oxford.

Blaxter, M. (1997) Whose fault is it? People's own conceptions of the reasons for health inequalities. *Social Science and Medicine*, **44**(6), 747–756.

Bowling, A. (1994) *Measuring Disease*, Open University Press, Buckingham.

Bowling, A. (1997) *Measuring Health*, 2nd edn, Open University Press, Buckingham.

Brannen, J. (1992) *Mixing Methods: Qualitative and Quantitative Research*, Avebury, Aldershot.

Brazier, J., Harper, R., Jones, N. *et al.* (1992) Validating the SF-36 health survey questionnaire: new outcome measure for primary care. *British Medical Journal*, **305**, 160–164.

Bruster, S., Jarman, B., Bosanquet, N. *et al.* (1994) National survey of hospital patients. *British Medical Journal*, **309**, 1542–1549.

Bryman, A. (1988) *Quantity and quality in social research*, Unwin Hyman, London.

Cartwright, A. (1983) *Health Surveys in Practice and Potential: A Critical Review of Their Scope and Methods*, King Edward's Hospital Fund for London, London.

Cartwright, A. and Seale, C. (1990) *A Natural History of a Survey*, King Edward's Hospital Fund for London, London.

Chambers, I. and Altman, D. (eds) (1995) *Systematic Reviews*, BMJ Publishing Group, London.

Charlton, J., Wallace, M. and White, I. (1994) Long-term illness: results from the 1991 Census. *Population Trends*, **75**.

Churchill, G. (1987) *Marketing Research – Methodological Foundations*, Holt, Rinehart & Winston, New York.

Clarke, G. and Cooke, D. (1992) *A Basic Course in Statistics*, Edward Arnold, Sevenoaks.

Cochran, W. (1954) Some methods for strengthening the common chi-square tests. *Biometrics*, **10**, 417–451.

Cox, B., Blaxter, M., Buckle, A. *et al.* (1987) *The Health and Lifestyle Survey*, Health Promotion Research Trust, London.

Crombie, I. with Davies, H. (1996) *Research in Health Care. Design, Conduct and Interpretation of Health Services Research*, John Wiley & Sons, Chichester.

Dale, A. and Marsh, C. (1993) *The 1991 Census User's Guide*, HMSO, London.

Dean, A., Dean, J., Coulombier, D. *et al.* (1995) *Epi Info, Version 6: A Word-Processing, Database, and Statistics Program for Public Health on IBM-compatible Computers.* Center for Disease Control and Prevention, Atlanta, GA.

Dixon, P. and Long, A. (1995) Broadening the criteria for selecting and developing health status instruments, in *Outcomes Briefing Issue 6, UK Clearing House on Health Outcomes*, Nuffield Institute for Health, Leeds.

Dowling, S., Barrett, S. and West, R. (1995) With nurse practitioners, who needs house officers? *British Medical Journal*, **311**, 309–313.

Eachus, J., Williams, M., Chan, P. *et al.* (1996) Deprivation and cause specific morbidity: evidence from the Somerset and Avon survey of health. *British Medical Journal*, **312**, 287–292.

Easterbrook, P., Berlin, J., Gopalan, R. and Matthews, D. (1991) Publication bias in clinical research. *Lancet*, **337**, 867–872.

Everitt, B. (1992) *The Analysis of Contingency Tables*, Chapman & Hall, London.

Fink, A. (1993) *Evaluation Fundamentals. Guiding health Programmes, Research and Policy*, Sage Publications, Newbury Park, CA.

Fink, A. (1995) *The Survey Handbook*, vol. 1, Sage Publications, Thousand Oaks, CA.

Fink, A. *et al.* (1995) *The Survey Kit*, (9 vols), Sage Publications, Thousand Oaks, CA.

Fitzpatrick, R. (1991a) Surveys of patient satisfaction: I – important general considerations. *British Medical Journal*, **302**, 887–889.

Fitzpatrick, R. (1991b) Surveys of patient satisfaction: II – designing a questionnaire and conducting a survey. *British Medical Journal*, **302**, 1129–1132.

Florey, C. du V. (1993) Sample size for beginners. *British Medical Journal*, **306**, 1181–1184.

Foddy, W. (1993) *Constructing Questions for Interviews and Questionnaires*, Cambridge University Press, Cambridge.

Forrest, R. and Gordon, D. (1995) *People and Places: A 1991 Census Atlas of England*, SAUS Publications, Bristol.

Fowler, F. (1993) *Survey Research Methods*, Sage Publications, Newbury Park, CA.

Gardner, M. and Altman, D. (eds) (1989) *Statistics with Confidence*, BMJ Publications, London.

Garratt, A., Ruta, D., Abdalla, M. and Russell, I. (1994) SF-36 health survey questionnaire: II. Responsiveness to changes in health status in four common clinical conditions. *Quality in Health Care*, **3**, 186–192.

Gerhardt, U. (1990) Qualitative research on chronic illness: the issue and the story. *Social Science and Medicine*, **30**, 11, 1149–1159.

Goffman, I. (1963) *Stigma: Notes on the Management of Spoiled Identity*, Penguin, Harmondsworth.

Gordon, D. and Forrest, R. (1995) *People and Places 2: Social and Economic Distinctions in England*, SAUS Publications, Bristol.

Greenhalgh, T. (1997a) Assessing the methodological quality of published papers. *British Medical Journal*, **315**, 305–308.

Greenhalgh, T. (1997b) Statistics for the non-statistician. II: "Significant' relations and their pitfalls. *British Medical Journal*, **315**, 422–425.

Haines, A. and Jones, R. (1994) Implementing findings of research. *British Medical Journal*, **308**, 1488–1492.

References

Hakim, C. (1987) *Research Design. Strategies and Choices in the Design of Social Research*, Allen & Unwin, London.

Hart, S. (1987) The use of the survey in industrial market research. *Journal of Marketing Management*, 3(1), 25–38.

Heurtin-Roberts, S. and Becker, G. (1993) Anthropological perspectives on chronic illness. *Social Science and Medicine*, 37(3), 281–283.

Hoare, J. (1992) *Tidal Wave: New Technology, Medicine and the NHS*, King's Fund, London.

Huff, D. (1973). *How to Lie with Statistics*, Penguin, Harmondsworth.

Hunter, D. (1993) Let's hear it for R&D. *Health Service Journal*, **15 Apr**, 17.

Illsley, R. and LeGrand, J. (1987) *Measurement and Inequality in Health*, Welfare State Programme Discussion Paper 12, London School of Economics, London.

Jenkinson, C., Layte, R., Wright, L. and Coulter, A. (1996) *The UK SF-36: An Analysis and Interpretation Manual*, Health Services Research Unit, University of Oxford, Oxford.

Jennett, B.(1988) Assessment of clinical technologies. Importance of provision and use. *International Journal of Technology Assessment in Health Care*, **4**, 435–445.

Jordan, K. (1996) *Limiting Long-term Illness: A Review of the Census Data and the Literature*, Centre for Health Planning and Management, Keele University, Keele.

Jordan, K., Croft, P. and Ong, B. N. (1997) *The Relationship Between General Practice Consultation and Reporting of a Limiting Long-term Illness*, Centre for Health Planning and Management and Industrial and Community Health Research Centre, Keele University, Keele.

Kanouse, D., Kallich, J. and Kahan, J. (1995) Dissemination of effectiveness and outcomes research. *Health Policy*, **34**, 167–192.

Ley, P. (1988) *Communicating With Patients. Improving Communication, Satisfaction and Compliance*, Croom Helm, London.

Lomas, J. and Haynes, R. (1988) A taxonomy and critical review of tested strategies for the application of clinical practice recommendations: from "official' to "individual' clinical policy. *American Journal of Preventive Medicine*, 4(4 Suppl.), 77–94.

Lwanga, S. and Lemeshow, S. (1991) *Sample Size Determination in Health Studies: A Practical Manual*, World Health Organization, Geneva.

Lyons, R., Lo, S. and Littlepage, B. (1994) Comparative health status of patients with 11 common illnesses in Wales. *Journal of Epidemiology and Community Health*, **48**, 388–390.

McAvoy, B. and Kaner, E. (1996) General practice postal surveys: a questionnaire too far? *British Medical Journal*, **313**, 732–733.

McDowell, I. and Jenkinson, C. (1996) Development standards for health measures. *Journal of Health Services Research and Policy*, **4**, 238–246.

McHorney, C., Kosinski, M. and Ware, J. (1994) Comparison of the costs and quality of norms for the SF-36 health survey collected by mail versus telephone interview results from a national survey. *Medical Care*, **32**, 551–567.

Malek, M. (1994) *Setting Priorities in Health Care*, John Wiley & Sons, Chichester.

Marsh, C. (1982) *The Survey Method: The Contribution of Surveys to Sociological Explanation*, Allen & Unwin, London.

Moore, D. (1991) *Statistics Concepts and Controversies*, W. H. Freeman, New York.

Moser, C. and Kalton, G. (1971) *Survey Methods in Social Investigation*, 2nd edn, Heinemann, London.

Ong, B. N. (1993) *The Practice of Health Services Research*, Chapman & Hall, London.

Ong, B. N., Jordan, K. and Richardson, J. (forthcoming) *The Experience of Limiting Long-standing Illness*.

Perneger T. (1998) What's wrong with Bonferroni adjustments. *British Medical Journal*, **316**, 1236–1238.

Petitti, D. (1994) *Meta-Analysis, Decision Analysis and Cost-Effectiveness Analysis*, Oxford University Press, New York.

Pett, M. (1997) *Nonparametric Statistics for Health Care Research*, Sage Publications, Thousand Oaks, CA.

Pocock, S. (1983) *Clinical Trials: A Practical Approach*, John Wiley & Sons, Chichester.

Rees, D (1994) *Essential Statistics for Medical Practice: A Case-Study Approach*, Chapman & Hall, London.

Sibbald, B., Addingtonhall, J., Brenneman, D. and Freeling, P. (1994) Telephone versus postal surveys of general practitioners methodological considerations. *British Journal of General Practice*

Siegel, S. and Castellan, N. (1988) *Nonparametric Statistics for the Behavioral Sciences*, McGraw-Hill, Singapore.

Snedecor, G. W. and Cochran, W. G. (1980) *Statistical Methods*, 7th edn, Iowa State University Press, Des Moines, IO.

Streiner, D. and Norman, G. (1995) *Health Measurement Scales – A Practical Guide to their Development and Use*, Oxford University Press, Oxford.

Sudman, S. and Bradburn, N. (1983) *Asking Questions: A Practical Guide to Questionnaire Design*, Jossey-Bass, San Francisco, CA.

Tufte, E. (1983) *The Visual Display of Quantitative Information*, Graphic Press, Cheshire, CT.

Ware, J., Snow, K., Kosinski, M. and Gandek, B. (1993) *SF-36 Health Survey Manual and Interpretation Guide*, Nimrod Press, Boston, MA.

WHO (1997) *The World Health Report 1997: Conquering Suffering, Enriching Humanity*, World Health Organization Office of World Health Reporting, Geneva.

Wilkin, D., Hallam, L. and Doggett, M. (1992) *Measures of Need and Outcome for Primary Health Care*, Oxford University Press, Oxford.

Williamson, I. and Whelan, T. (1996) The clinical problem of Bell's palsy: is treatment with steroids effective? *British Journal of General Practice*, **46**, 743–747.

Wright, D. (1997) *Understanding Statistics: An Introduction for the Social Sciences*, Sage Publications, London.

INDEX

Index